Raising D

MW01223652

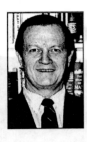

About the Author

Dr. Bruce Miller's postgraduate studies at New York University included clinical, nutrition oriented research which focused on nutrition problems of the elderly.

Dr. Miller is a member of the Linus Pauling Institute of Science Medicine, a charter member of Dr. Kenneth Cooper's Aerobics Center, a member of the International Academy of Preventive Medicine, International College of Applied Nutrition, founder of the Diet Analysis Center, and a consultant to the American Running and Fitness Association.

Dr. Miller is a Certified Nutrition Specialist and a member of the American College of Nutrition. Currently Dr. Miller is the Director of Research for the American Academy of Nutrition. Dr. Miller lives in Dallas with Jody, his wife of more than 40 years.

Published in arrangement with Oak Publications Sdn Bhd.

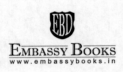
www.embassybooks.in

Published in India by :
EMBASSY BOOKS,
120 Great Western Building,
M.C. C. Lane, Kala Ghoda, Fort,
Mumbai - 400 023.
Tel : +9122 22819546 / 32967415
Email : info@embassybooks.in
www.embassybooks.in

ISBN : 978-93-83359-85-1

Chapter 1

Inculcate
Healthy Eating Habits
from Young

Parents are mostly caught up with wanting their children to be top performers in their studies, sometimes at the expense of their health. There is nothing wrong in wanting children to perform well academically, but it is also equally important to give priority to their health at the same time. "Neither Rome nor a healthy lifestyle can be built in a day. Developing a healthy lifestyle requires consistency, not perfection," says Dr. Gordon Tessler.

Healthy eating habits are an important ingredient in raising healthy disease free kids. Dr McDougall, in his book, *Digestive Tune-up* aptly says, "The food you put into your body is the single most powerful factor that determines your health and well-being."

It is very important to inculcate the right eating habits during your children's formative years. Once they are able to feed themselves, it will very difficult for you to make changes to their eating habits. The habits formed while they are young will probably be with them for life. "Bad habits are easier to abandon today than tomorrow," says a Jewish proverb.

CHALLENGING TIMES FOR PARENTS

Most parents today are finding it challenging to inculcate

healthy eating habits in their children. We are now a nation of speed eaters and grazers. Rarely do we sit down with the entire family to have three healthy home-cooked meals a day.

Today, what our children eat daily is largely directed by huge food companies with their monstrous advertising budget. If the food manufacturers can train your child to eat their products, then that child's buying and eating habits will continue into adulthood. The number of overweight and undernourished children in the United States has more than doubled since the 1960s, bears witness to this fact.

More younger children than ever before are being diagnosed with diseases related to lifestyle and diet such as pre-diabetes, pre-hypertension, cancer, and heart disease; all unrelated to germs. Most of these diseases have their roots in childhood.

Changing Diets

Our diets have changed drastically. In fact, our diets have changed more in the last 30 years than they did in the previous hundred years. The foods you are eating today are over-processed, grease-soaked, sugar-filled, and chemical-laden, as compared to the fresh whole foods your ancestors ate.

Through pasteurization, homogenization, high heat, and mechanical processing, your foods are deprived of its nutrients to such an extent that your food has to be "enriched" by artificially adding back some of the nutrients lost. This is especially true of white flour where some vitamins are added back after the processing is done. The more processing a food goes through, the more nutrient value it loses.

Chemical Additives

There are more than 3,000 direct and indirect common chemical additives present in our diet; nearly two-thirds of them are flavorings used to replace the natural flavors lost during processing.

The food processors begin with white flour, sugar, fat, and water. By the use of flavors, colors, and texturing chemicals they can produce just about any taste they want. The simple "potato chip" is a good example. The processors start with a nice healthy potato. After they finish destroying over 95 percent of the nutrients, they then add fat (trans fatty acids), sugar (refined or artificial sweeteners) and refined salt to it.

The great majority of these food additives have absolutely nothing to do with nutritional value. The object of the additives is to develop new foods, to enhance consumer acceptability, and to feed our illusions about what looks and tastes healthy. To improve the shelf life of certain products, processors embalm them. Bread has sixteen chemicals to keep it "fresh."

Besides chemical additives, pesticides are also found in our vegetables and fruits, while our meat and dairy products are tainted with antibiotics and growth hormones.

Junk and Instant Foods

Multimedia advertising is possibly the most dangerous assault to your children's health in America today! Sad to say, but most parents and children get their nutritional information from television and the mass media. Commercial products advertised in the mass media are mostly high in sugar, fat and salt.

Junk food contains high levels of saturated fat, salt, sugar, chemical additives, flavorings, and preservatives. At the same time, they also lacking in proteins, vitamins and fibers. Manufacturers favor producing junk food because it's relatively cheap to produce; it has a long shelf life and it does not need refrigeration.

It is popular with consumers because it is convenient, requires little or no preparation and it is tasty. Consumption of junk food is associated with obesity, heart disease, Type 2 diabetes and dental cavities.

Besides the mass media and the manufacturers of refined foods, many parents are at fault for not providing healthy meals for themselves and their children. Juggling busy schedules, household chores, school and extra-curricular activities seem to be some of the common reasons. The result:

We want convenience which means ease of preparation. The traditional sit-down, relaxed family dinner has gone the way of fast or "quick to cook" processed food products.

Children are surrounded by fast-food outlets in schools, soda and candy machines, and junky snacks in classrooms and at parties, parades, holiday celebrations, and just about everywhere else.

Healthy nutritious foods have been replaced by the following four groups: Fast food (microwaveable and pre-cooked), frozen foods, fatty foods and fake foods.

Under the above circumstances, it is indeed challenging for parents today to bring up disease free children. However, this challenge is surmountable and that is what this book is all about.

MEETING THE CHALLENGE

So what can we do? We can meet the challenges of this changing diet by instilling in your children healthy eating habits from childhood. Developing children's attitude towards food is like teaching your children how to handle money and allowing them to make sensible choices and be responsible for their decisions.

Healthy eating represents a lifestyle, which involves balanced, nutritious meals to be eaten at least three times a day. As parents your role is to guide them down the right path.

Below are some manageable changes, you may want to use to create an environment that encourages your child to develop good eating habits:

- Make a game of reading food labels. The whole family will learn what's good for their health and be more conscious of what they eat. Briefly, here are some of the things you need to look for in the label: The serving size, the number of calories in the food, the kind of fat, sodium content, dietary fiber, sugars, proteins, vitamins and minerals and the presence of chemical additives.

- Make a wide variety of nutritious foods available to your children instead of refined foods or junk foods. All healthy nutritious foods contain different levels of vitamins, minerals and nutrients. Just make junk or highly processed foods a rare treat and healthy foods a way of life.

- Be a positive role model. If you're practicing healthy habits, it"'s a lot easier to convince your children to do the same. Children are intelligent and they can learn very quickly to emulate your good or bad habits.

- Try not to use food to punish or reward your children.

- Encourage your children to eat slowly. Give plenty of time for them to enjoy their meals.

- Involve your children in shopping, preparing and cooking meals. These activities will give you the opportunity to impart to your children how to develop healthy eating habits. As a result, your children may be more willing to eat or try foods that they help prepare.

- Make sure your children's meals outside the home are balanced or in case of doubts, pack their lunch to include a variety of foods.

- Don't forget to select healthier items when dining at restaurants.

- Limit the amount of salt and sugar in your child's diet. Replace refined sugar or artificial sweeteners with natural sugars and refined salt with unrefined salt.

- To prevent your children from over eating at lunch or at snack time, make sure your child takes his breakfast. Studies have shown that children who eat breakfast do better at school.

- Get in the habit of offering water over juice concentrates. Over consumption of sweetened drinks and sodas are associated with obesity in children.

- Educate them on the nutrients present in fruits and vegetables and how they play a role in their growing years.

- Never force your children to eat or finish all their food. Fighting and yelling at your children will only make them resent the food more. If they disobey, politely tell them that they cannot snack later on or offer them a healthy snack instead.

- Make mealtimes a family event where the whole family eats together.

- For your children to know more about the nutritional values of vegetables and fruits, teach them how to start a garden and tend to it.

- Educate your children about the dangers of eating disorders such anorexia and bulimia.

PUTTING IT TOGETHER

Take the advice of John A. McDougall, a well known medical doctor and author of McDonald Medicine, "Diet and lifestyle are the causes of most deaths and disabilities that people suffer in the United States today."

Do not take your children's health for granted nor place

the health of your children to someone else. Diseases develop, it doesn't start overnight. Parents should not start working on their children's health until they are faced with a crisis.

Practice prevention rather than treat disease in order to bring up disease free kids. Prevention is about taking steps while you are healthy. It is much easier to prevent a killer disease before it happens than to try to regain health once it has taken its toll. Killer diseases like cancer, diabetes, heart attack, stroke, all have their roots in childhood.

I would like to end this chapter with this parting message to parents and would be parents that, "Health is like money, we never have a true idea of its value until we lose it." Most people will only realize the value of health when they lose it. They will then pay any cost to recover from their illness. Don't be like these people.

GOLD NUGGETS

"Train up a child in the way he should go: And when he is old, he will not depart from it." – Proverbs

"An unfortunate thing about this world is that the good habits are much easier to give up than the bad ones." – W. Somerset Maugham

"When it comes to eating right and exercising, there is no I will start tomorrow. Tomorrow is disease." – V.L. Allineare

"Good habits formed at youth make all the difference." – Aristotle

"We first make our habits, and then our habits make us." – John Dryden

"If we're not willing to settle for junk living, we certainly shouldn't settle for junk food." – Sally Edwards

"The patient should be made to understand that he or she must take charge of his own life. Don't take your body to the doctor as if he were a repair shop." – Quentin Regestein

"Children need models rather than critics." – Joseph Joubert

"Children are apt to live up to what you believe of them." – Lady Bird Johnson.

"Children have never been very good at listening to their elders, but they have never failed to imitate them." – James Baldwin.

"Your children will see what you're all about by what you live rather than what you say." – Dr. Wayne Dyer.

"The quality, not the longevity, of one's life is what is important." – Martin Luther King Jr.

"To bring up a child in the way he should go, travel that way yourself once in a while." – Josh Billings.

"Your children need your presence more than your presents." – Jesse Jackson.

"Don't worry that children never listen to you, worry that they are always watching you." – Robert Fulham.

"Procrastination is opportunity's natural assassin." – Victor Kiam

"If you don't like something change it; if you can't change it, change the way you think about it." – Mary Engelbret

"Our greatest weakness lies in giving up. The most certain way to succeed is always to try just one more time." – Thomas Edison

Chapter 2

Think Fruits and Vegetables

Researchers from Johns Hopkins University confirm that Americans are not getting better at eating fruits and vegetables. The Johns Hopkins study shows that, among U.S. adults, fruit consumption is holding steady, but vegetable consumption is headed down. The study appeared in the *American Journal of Preventive Medicine.*

The U.S. Department of Agriculture (USDA) Food Guide Pyramid recommends 2-4 servings of fruits and 3-5 servings of vegetables each day. In my opinion, this is the absolute minimum children should be eating.

NUTRITIONAL VALUE

Fruits and vegetables should make up a large portion of your children's diet. They are low in calories, high in vitamins, minerals, phytochemicals (plant nutrients), antioxidants, enzymes and fiber. They help boost your child's immune system, the body's first line of defense against "foreign invaders."

A weak immune system can leave your children open to all kinds of diseases as the immune system incorporates the body's total response to illness. From recognition of early warning signs to full-scale battle, the immune system is the main barrier against any disease.

Phytochemicals

Dr. Brenda Davis, writing in her book *Defeating Diabetes*, describes phytochemicals as, immune-enhancing, anti-inflammatory, anti-viral, anti-bacterial, anti-fungal, anti-yeast and anti-motion sickness.

In the past few years, there has been an explosion of research on phytochemicals. These are constituents of various plants, mostly carotenoids and flavonoids that have powerful antioxidant properties.

Carotenoids

The carotenoids are a family of plant pigments with at least 700 members. About 60 of them are found in commonly eaten foods. They provide the reds, oranges, yellows and other colors of the rainbow. Lycopene, lutein, zeaxanthin and beta carotene are the better known of the carotenoid family.

Flavonoids

Flavonoids are the umbrella term given to some 4000 compounds that are found in plants, notably in the pigments of leaves, barks, rinds, seeds and flowers. Two well known flavonoids are quercetin and proanthocyandins (OPC). They are also found in beverages like green tea, black tea and red wine.

Flavonoids have been studied since the 1940s, and their antioxidant activity is totally undisputed. With the immense volume of research being released every year expanding on the actions of flavonoids, more and more scientists are becoming convinced that optimal intake of flavonoids is essential for disease prevention, treatment and vibrant health.

Flavonoids and carotenoids complement each other in that they each target different cells, tissues and organs. The flavonoids being water soluble, works in the watery part of the membrane, whereas carotenoids being oil soluble, works in the oily part of the cell membrane.

Sources of Phytochemicals
Choosing a wide variety of colorful, whole plant foods is the key to a phytochemical-rich diet. Here are an array of vegetables and fruits of the rainbow color that are rich in phytochemicals:

Red: Tomato, watermelon, pink guava and grapefruit contain lycopene, a member of the carotenoid family, that prevents abnormal growth of cells and strengthen heart functions to protect against heart disease.

Red purple: Grapes, blueberries, blackberries, beetroot and strawberries contain anthocyanidin, a powerful antioxidant that improves circulation to the eyes and protects the health of the blood vessels against heart disease.

Orange: Carrots, sweet potatoes, pumpkin, mango and winter squash contain beta-carotene which helps to boost immune function and protect against breast cancer.

Orange-yellow: Oranges, tangerines, peaches, pine-apples and nectarines, are high in vitamin C, a powerful cell protector.

Orange-green: Spinach, kale, green beans, yellow corn, turnip, mustard or collard green containing lutein that protects the health of your eyes.

Green: Cruciferous vegetables such as broccoli, brussel sprouts, cabbage, bok choy, cauliflower, containing sulforaphane, isthiocynate and indole that have powerful cancer properties.

White-green: Garlic, onions, chives, leeks and shallots contains sulphur compounds that helps protect your DNA. Asparagus, peas, mushrooms, and celery contain flavonoids that protect cell membranes from free radicals.

Antioxidants

Antioxidants are a group of compounds that are produced by the body and are also found naturally in plant foods. They are the police force of your body that defends your healthy cells and tissues from free radicals.

Free radicals are incomplete, unstable molecules. They are like a shark feeding frenzy. They rip, tear and damage that which they attack. They cause cut apples and potatoes to turn brown and fatty meats to turn rancid. Antioxidants act as scavengers to prevent cell and tissue damage from free radicals that could lead you down the road to many degenerative diseases.

Vitamins and Minerals

Fruits and vegetables are also rich in: Beta-carotene, vitamin C and vitamin E. They also provide various amounts of vitamin B and a very rich source of minerals like calcium, potassium, iron, selenium, phosphorus and protein.

Enzymes

Virtually all uncooked fruits and vegetables are good sources of enzymes. According to Dr. Edward Howell, the father of food enzyme therapy, enzymes are, "Substances that make life possible; they are the spark of life. No mineral or vitamin can do any work without enzymes. They are the manual workers that build your body from proteins, carbohydrates, and fats. Without the life energy of enzymes, we would be nothing more than a pile of lifeless chemical substances – vitamins, minerals, water and proteins."

We are not only what we eat, but what is digested and assimilated that keeps us healthy and energetic. Good digestion is one of the foundations of good health. Without enzymes, proper digestion cannot occur, our cells would not receive adequate nutrition and our health is compromised. Enzymes may be the key to defying disease and extending the life of your children.

Fiber

Your children need fiber from fruits and vegetables to keep their digestive system running smoothly to eliminate wastes regularly, and reduce the incidence of constipation. Fibers also protect them from heart disease, high blood pressure, excess blood fats and prevent cancer of the colon. Fiber can help control appetite and help you lose weight.

Fiber is only found in plants. The dietary fibers are classified as soluble or insoluble. The National Institute of Cancer recommends a daily consumption of 25 to 30 grams of fiber daily.

Soluble fibers dissolve in water, soaking up fluid in your stomach and small intestine. It works like a 'sponge,' slowing the absorption of your food. That's what gives you that full, satisfied feeling after a meal and therefore, discourages overeating. Soluble fibers can help lower cholesterol, lower blood pressure, and lower triglycerides.

Insoluble fiber is not a "sponge" but a "broom." It moves through your body fairly quickly, sweeping out wastes, toxins, poisons, and potential cancer causing chemicals before your body can absorb them.

Since water insoluble fibers absorb water, it is important to get your children to drink plenty of liquids along with increased dietary fiber intake. Increasing fiber too rapidly can initially cause excess gas formation or diarrhea.

The more highly processed or refined a food and the more instant its preparation, the lower its fiber and nutrient content.

Sources of Fiber

Whole grains cereals: By whole grain, we mean the entire cereal grain which consists of three layers – the bran, the germ, and the endosperm. Most of the grains we consume are refined cereals, where the three layers mentioned above have been removed. Refined grains looks polished and white, with 80 percent of its nutrients lost. Whole grain cereals include: Brown, wild and basmati rice, barley, corn, wheat, and oats.

Seeds and nuts: Almonds, chestnuts, lotus seeds, peanuts, pumpkin seeds, sesame seeds, sunflower seeds, and walnuts.

Beans: Red beans, broad beans, black-eyed beans, chick peas, lentils, mung beans, peas, and soybeans.

Soy products: Tempeh and miso.

INCREASE YOUR CHILD'S VEGETABLE INTAKE

Getting kids to eat fruits is usually not a problem but getting them to eat especially vegetables is a challenge for many parents. Busy school schedules and the temptation of junk foods are some barriers to getting enough fruits and vegetables into your children's diet. Want your kids to eat their veggies? Here are a few ways that may help:

- One of the best ways to get children interested in eating vegetables is to start a garden at home, so they can eat the vegetables they grow. Have your child harvest the vegetables and cook it at the next meal. This will give them the opportunity to learn more about the vegetables and its nutritional values.

- Start putting vegetables on your children's plate as early as possible.

- Research shows that if you let your children pick the vegetables they want to eat when you go shopping; they are more likely to enjoy eating them.

- Set a good example. Children are more likely to eat a variety of vegetables if they see their parents eating and enjoying them.

- Always include vegetables at meals and snacks. Offer a

variety and prepare them in different ways.

- Research shows that it can take 8-15 tries of a new food before your child accepts it. Often parents stop offering a new food after 3 to 5 tries, so don't give up easily.

- Make mealtimes fun and don't try to force your kids to eat things they don't want.

- Look for creative ways to offer your kids vegetables. Try making vegetable smoothies or make designs out of vegetables for their snacks and meals.

- If children are old enough, let them help chop, clean, peel, or cut up fruits and vegetables. Kids usually eat the dishes that they help, select and prepare.

HOW TO CHOOSE VEGETABLES?

As vegetables are perishable, don't buy more than you need. The amount of nutrients lost in vegetables depends on the length of time they are exposed to air, heat and water.

Look for ones that look crisp with no signs of wilting. If the vegetable is fresh, the leaf rib should snap sharply.

For root vegetables such as potatoes and onions, choose those that are firm, free of bruises, holes or cut. If you are concerned about harmful chemicals like pesticides in vegetables, you may opt to go organic. Organically grown vegetables have a higher nutrient content than conventionally grown ones. However, if you are concerned about chemicals in conventional grown vegetables, consider buying an ozone 3 detoxifier.

GOLD NUGGETS

"If slaughterhouses had glass walls, everyone would be a vegetarian." – Paul McCartney.

"I don't understand why asking people to eat a well-balanced vegetarian diet is considered drastic, while it is medically conservative to cut people open." – Dean Ornish, M.D.

"Life expectancy would grow by leaps and bounds if green vegetables smelled as good as bacon." – Author unknown.

"Adopting a new healthier lifestyle can involve changing diet to include more fresh fruit and vegetables as well as increasing levels of exercise." – Linford Christie.

Chapter 3

Feed Them
with the Right Fats

Fats and oils have a direct and profound impact on the health of your children. We have been often told again and again in the mass media that fats are bad for health because they are associated with degenerative diseases such as heart disease, cancer and diabetes. This has made many of us switch from butter (saturated fats) to margarine (trans fatty acids) as a better alternative. Are we really moving in the right direction?

To provide some answers, I am going to unravel some truth about fats and why eating the right fats early in your children's life can prevent the very diseases that fats are claimed to be responsible for.

THE TRUTH ABOUT FATS

First Truth: A Low Fat No Fat Diet Is Dangerous.

According to Dr. Udo Erasmus, a world authority on fats and oil, "A no fat diet over a long period will kill you and a low fat diet will make you ill. The low fat (no fat) diet that is the rage today leads to stunted growth in children; dry skin; low energy levels; high cholesterol; high triglycerides; compromised immune function; leaky gut and allergies; lower testosterone production. It is far more important to bring in the good fats than to avoid the bad fats. A low fat, no fat diet take us in the wrong direction, what we need is a right fat approach."

Second Truth: Fats Do Not Make You Fat.
Fats do not make you fat. In fact, we should be eating more fats. Fats suppress appetite. Most problems involving excess weight are due to excessive intake of sweet and starchy foods that are high in glycemic index and glycemic load, accompanied by a sedentary lifestyle.

Certain fats, especially the essential fatty acids (EFA) help us lose body fat. EFAs increase body fat burning and decrease body fat production and increase heat production (burn off fat without exercise).

Third Truth: We Need the Right Fats.
Just as there are good and bad cholesterol, similarly there are "good" and "bad" fats. "There are good fats that are absolutely required for health and bad fats that are harmful to your children's health. What we need is not a high fat, low, no fat or fake fat diet. What we need is the *right fat diet*. These are essential fatty acids that your body can't produce and that you must get from your diet," says Dr. Udo Erasmus.

Fourth Truth: Fats Are Vital To Your Health.
Fatty acids are the building blocks of fats, much like amino acids are the building blocks of proteins. Fats make up at least 50 percent of the cell membranes, making it permeable so that nutrients can get into the cell and waste material can be removed from the cell, keep the skin soft and supple and help premature wrinkling of the skin.

Throughout life, fat is essential to provide energy and support growth. Fats contain nine calories per gram as compared to four calories per gram from protein and carbohydrates. During infancy and childhood, fat – a macro-nutrient – is necessary for normal brain development.

Fats help absorb fat soluble vitamins such as A, D, E and K. Dietary fats are needed for the conversion of beta carotene to vitamin A. Fats help keep the body warm. They are also building blocks of hormones and they insulate the nervous system tissue in the body.

Fifth Truth: Low Fat Foods Are Not Healthy.

Low fat foods are not tasty because fats enhance taste. To overcome the problem of taste; many manufacturers load low fat foods with sugar, which your body turns into hard (saturated) fats. So instead of your food being loaded with fats you are now loaded with sugar – another health killer.

Sixth Truth: There Is No Established RDA For Fats.

Although there is no RDA for fats, most health authorities recommend people to limit fats to 25-30 percent of their caloric intake, which is about 2½ ounces or 5 tablespoons per day for a diet of 2400 calories.

THE GOOD FATS

All fats are not created equal. To understand how fat affects health, it is necessary to understand the different types of fats available and the ways in which these fats act within the body.

The good fats and oils in nutrition are called essential fatty acids from polyunsaturated fats that are needed by every living cell in your body. Your body cannot make them and so it must come from your food. The two essential fatty acids your children need are the omega-3 fatty acids and the omega-6 fatty acids.

Omega-3 Fatty Acids

Eicosapentaenoic Acid (EPA), an omega-3 fatty acid, is one of the structural components in cell walls and membranes of the body. The cell membrane allows nutrients to enter the cell and ensures that waste products are removed quickly. Cells without a healthy membrane lose their ability to hold water and vital nutrients. EPA produces a membrane with a high degree of integrity and fluidity.

EPA is extremely beneficial to the heart: Helps to prevent blood clots caused by platelet aggregation (clumping together), cause dilation (opening) of blood vessels and keep blood vessels wide open, and keeps the blood flowing freely.

The Food and Drug Administration gave "qualified health claim" status to EPA and docosahexaenoic acid (DHA) stating that, "Supportive but not conclusive research shows that consumption of EPA and DHA fatty acids may reduce the risk of coronary heart disease."

EPA not only can help lower serum cholesterol but it can also improve the ratio of HDL to LDL which helps you reduce your risk of a heart attack. Omega-3 fatty acids may also help lower triglycerides. Several other studies also suggest that these fatty acids may help lower high blood pressure.

Fish oils also contain DHA. DHA is crucial for brain function. The human brain is one of the largest "consumers" of DHA. A normal adult human brain contains more than 20 grams of DHA. Research shows that low DHA levels are associated with depression, suicide, and violence.

You can get EPA and DHA from cold water fish such as salmon, herring, tuna, cod and mackerel. It is also available from flaxseed but this source is not as effective.

You can source EPA from nuts (hazelnuts, almonds, pecans, cashews, walnuts, and macadamia nuts) and from dark green leafy vegetables, soybean, flaxseed oil and canola oil.

Omega-6 Fatty Acids

Gamma linolenic acid (GLA) is the most important omega-6 fatty acid of the linoleic acid family. The main source of GLA is found in mother's milk, the oils of evening primrose and borage. The body can also convert linoleic acid into GLA but as we age, our bodies become less efficient at converting linoleic acid to GLA. For this reason most nutritionists recommend taking GLA as a supplement.

GLA is also known to help people with skin problems, obesity, rheumatoid arthritis, heart disease, high blood pressure.

Most of these ailments affect us, as we age.

Balance Is Critical
American diets are overloaded with Omega-6 fatty acids and deficient in Omega-3 fatty acids. Your body needs both fats but we need them in balance. Too much of one or the other can cause a variety of health problems in the body.

Omega-9 Fatty Acids
Omega-9 fatty acids, also called oleic acid are derived from monounsaturated fats. Oleic acid is important for heart health, as it works by increasing HDL levels in the body, and helps to reduce LDLs in the blood, although it is not an essential fatty acid. However, new research shows it has a role in keeping us healthy. Foods with omega-9 fatty acids include olives and olive oil, most nuts, and avocados.

THE BAD FATS

Saturated Fats
Saturated fats are usually solid at room temperature, and they're more stable as they don't combine readily with oxygen. This means that they do not normally turn rancid, even when heated for cooking purposes.

Saturated fats in the typical American diet, comes mainly from animal sources such as dairy products like whole milk, butter and cheese cream and from fatty meats like beef, veal, pork, lamb and lard.

The liver uses saturated fats to manufacture cholesterol. Therefore, excessive dietary intake of saturated fats by your children can significantly raise the blood cholesterol level, especially the level of low-density lipoproteins (LDLs), the "bad cholesterol."

Eating a diet rich in red meat has been linked to an increased risk of cardiovascular disease and some cancers. Since red meat has the highest concentration of saturated fats, many experts suggest that you limit your children's consumption of red meat to only two or three small servings per week.

THE UGLY FATS

Most of the health problems that we blame on fats should be blamed on the destructive processing to which fats have been subjected to. There are three ways oil processing methods turn good fats to ugly fats: Hydrogenation, refining and deep frying.

Hydrogenation

Trans fatty acids (trans fat or hydrogenated fats) are created during a process called *hydrogenation* when food manufacturers add heat, pressure and hydrogen gas to unsaturated vegetable oils to turn it into solid or semi solid fats. "Hydrogenate" means to add hydrogen. Hydrogenation can be either fully or partially hydrogenated.

Hydrogenation is the most common way of drastically changing natural polyunsaturated oils to 'synthetic' or man-made fats. Hydrogenation ruins the nutritional value of vegetable oils. It was invented as an alternative to saturated fats. Butter and lard being saturated fats were replaced by margarine and vegetable shortenings.

When liquid oil is partially hydrogenated, the resulting fat is laden with trans fatty acids. Fatty acids are the building block of fats, much like amino acids are the building blocks of protein.

The partially hydrogenated fats are ideal for frying and commercial baking because of its high melting point, its creamy, smooth texture and its reusability in deep-fat frying but at the expense of your health. Hydrogenation, not only extends the shelf life of a product such as cookies, cakes, fries and doughnuts but it also gives them a less greasy feeling.

In short: Hydrogenated oils can be called 'white' oils and are equivalent to refined (white) sugar. Like sugar, they are nutrient-deficient sources of calories but unlike sugar they contain toxins.

What Do Researchers Say About Trans Fatty Acids?
"Numerous studies have found that trans fatty acids raise our risk of heart disease. They can also contribute to an increase in Total cholesterol levels and a drop in the healthy HDL cholesterol. These man-made fats are much worse for you than any other natural fat, even the saturated fats found in butter and beef." said Mary Beth Sodus, a registered dietitian at the University of Maryland Medical Center.

Dr, Joanne Lunn of the British Nutrition Foundation has this to say about the negative effects of trans fats, "They have being shown not only to raise LDL cholesterol in the blood but also to lower HDL cholesterol. In other words, like saturated fats, trans fats also raise LDL cholesterol but unlike saturated fats, they also simultaneously lower HDL cholesterol."

"Trans fatty acids can increase blood cholesterols by up to 15 percent and blood fats (triglycerides) levels by up to 47 percent very rapidly when partially hydrogenated vegetable oil containing 37 percent fatty acids is ingested. High triglyceride levels play a part in developing cardiovascular disease. If your diet contains cholesterol, the effect of trans fatty acid is enhanced," says Dr. Udo Uramus, author of *Fats That Heal and Fats That Kill.*

Siegfried Gursche, founder of the *Alive* magazine in Canada, calls trans fatty acids, "The single most dangerous ingredient in our food. Trans fatty acids are so heavily processed, they aren't even food any more. They're like plastic. The molecular structure of the oil is so damaged by hydrogenation that the liver doesn't even recognize it as food. It can't digest trans fatty acid and tries to flush them out of our system by producing more cholesterol. That's where our high cholesterol levels come from."

According to Stephen Joseph, founder of bantransfats.com, "Trans fatty acids are put into food products to increase shelf life, but they shorten human life. Trans fatty acids are not edible food."

Researchers at the Harvard School of Public Health and the Wageningen Centre for Food Sciences in the Netherlands took a look at 25 studies on the subject and concluded, in the prestigious New England Journal of Medicine, that the more trans fatty acids you eat, the higher your risk of a coronary disease.

The Harvard University's Nurse's Health Study of 85,000 US women, found a 53 percent increase in risk of heart disease in those who ate the most trans fatty acids; compared with those who ate the least.

Similarly, a study published in 1997 by the *New England Journal of Medicine* claimed that eating just one gram of trans fatty acids a day, increased a person's chance of developing cardiovascular disease by 20 percent.

Is Your Children's Food Safe from Trans Fatty Acids?
They wouldn't put hydrogenated fats in your kids' foods, right? Wrong! Kid's foods have some of the highest levels of hydrogenated fats and children are the last people who should be eating hydrogenated fats. Fast food is loaded with trans fatty acids. Their hamburgers, hot dog buns, French fries and fried chicken are mostly fried in pure hydrogenated fat. However, things are changing for the better as most fast food chains are starting to find a better alternative to trans fats.

Trans fats are also high in breakfast cereals, cookies and crackers, breakfast bars, snack bars, peanut butter, pancake mixes, instant soups, chocolate, desserts, fruit cakes, chips, convenience and junk foods, peanut butter, some salad dressings, margarine, most refined cooking oils, salads oil, mayonnaise, vegetable shortening and fried foods.

Learn To Read Food Labels
The following fancy words on food labels indicate the presence of trans fatty acids: Zero trans fats, hydrogenated vegetable oil, partially hydrogenated vegetable oil, vegetable shortenings, cholesterol free, cooked in vegetable oils, low in saturated fat,

made with 100 percent vegetable oil, vegetable oil and fat or even vegetable margarine. Wow! Can't imagine you can skin a cat in so many ways.

Refining

High heat – as well as exposure to light and oxygen – turns oil rancid. Most oil sold in your super or hyper market, grocery or convenience stores whether from safflower, soybean, canola, peanut or other nut sources are fully refined and deodorized and are either solvent-extracted or a mixture of expeller-pressed and solvent extracted oils. All these oils are colorless, odorless and tasteless. You can find selling information such as "free of cholesterol," "high in polyunsaturates," and "low in saturates for frying, baking and cooking" on labels of refined oils.

Modern commercial oils are sold in see-through plastic bottles because they had already turned rancid and gone through refining, bleaching and deodorization to mask the rancidity. This is why unrefined oils are traditionally stored in dark bottles, in cool places.

Refined oils are the equivalent to refined (white) sugars, and can be called "white oil." They are devoid of most minerals, vitamins, protein, fiber, lecithin and phytosterols.

Rancid oils are very toxic. They are as harmful as trans fatty acids, or possibly even more harmful. Refining oils introduces toxic molecules, resulting from the breakdown and alteration of fatty acid molecules.

Even though they may not contain trans fats, such oils contain lots of free radicals, which can cause serious damage to the cells of the body. Many lipid experts believe that, apart from trans fatty acids, rancid oils are another major cause of heart disease, cancer and other degenerative diseases.

Deep Frying

Oils in transparent bottles are rich in the essential fatty acids becomes toxic when fried above 160 degree C. The burnt parts of fried, deep-fried, toasted, roasted, baked, broiled, barbecued foods are toxic.

In commercial deep frying, the same batch of oil is often kept at high temperature constantly for days. They contain many toxic substances that have been proven harmful to the human body. They could be more toxic than trans fatty acids.

So what is the best oil for frying? If health is what you have in mind for your children, water is the only oil appropriate for frying. We're back to steaming, poaching, boiling, or pressure cooking our foods.

If you want to use fats for deep frying, use saturated fats for frying as they are the least damaging. They include coconut oil, palm oil, and butter in small quantities. However, very high heat can also turn saturated fats into many toxic substances.

CHOLESTEROL

Dr. Kenneth Cooper aptly says, "A very important part of preventing heart attacks is controlling your cholesterol – not eliminating it all together."

We cannot eliminate cholesterol from our diet completely. Cholesterol builds and repair cells. It is part of all cell membranes. It is used to produce our sex hormones and it is converted into bile acids in the body to help digest fats.

Cholesterol comes mainly from animal sources. The safe range intake is between 200 to 400 milligrams per day.

You need to lower the LDL cholesterol, the bad cholesterol and increase HDL cholesterol in the blood. Excess bad cholesterol is widely accepted as the best indicator of the rate your arteries are aging.

Excess bad cholesterol can cause: Aging of coronary arteries, plaque buildup, a heart attack, and stroke. For more detailed information on cholesterol, please read my book, *7 Keys to Normalize Your Cholesterol Level.*

Food Sources	Cholesterol per 100 g of food in mg
Beef – loin, raw	70
Beef – on average, raw	59
Beef – ribs, raw	58
Beef – tongue, raw	108
Butter – ordinary	220
Bone marrow	3000
Camembert cheese – whole fat	73
Caviar	50
Cheddar cheese – whole fat	90
Chicken – breast, meat only, raw	64
Chicken – dark meat, meat only, raw	83
Chicken – liver, raw	380
Chicken eggs – whole, raw	600
Chicken eggs – yolk, raw	1790
Cod – smoked	50
Cod-liver oil	850
Cottage cheese – whole fat	37
Cream – 20 percent fat	66
Cream – 35 percent fat	120
Dried milk – powder, whole fat	109
Duck – on average, raw	76
Edam cheese – fat	71
Emmentaler cheese – fat	83
Goose – on average, raw	80
Hen – on average, raw	81
Herring – raw	64
Herring in oil	52
Herring in tomato sauce	50
Horse – on average, meat only, raw	75
Ice-cream	34
Kefir – natural, 2 percent fat	8
Lard	95

Mackerel – smoked	70
Meat paté	130
Milk – cow, 3,5 percent fat	14
Milk – goat	11
Milk – sheep	27
Mutton – leg, raw	78
Mutton – meat only, raw	78
Perch – raw	38
Pork – belly, raw	60
Pork – ham, raw	60
Pork – hearts, raw	140
Pork – kidney, raw	375
Pork – loin, raw	69
Pork – liver, raw	300
Pork – on average, raw	61
Pork – spare ribs, raw	66
Pork fat	99
Pork sausage	100
Rabbit – on average, raw	65
Salmon – raw	360
Sardines in oil	120
Shrimps – raw	152
Trout – raw	55
Tuna in oil	55
Turkey – breast, meat and skin, raw	65
Turkey – dark meat, meat and skin, raw	72
Turkey – on average	68
Veal – leg, raw	71
Veal – meat only, raw	71
Veal brain	2830
Yogurt – natural, 2 percent fat	8

PUTTING IT TOGETHER

Manufacturers are now introducing new, low fat margarines as trans-free. Oil processors are mixing super-hard, trans-free hydrogenated oils with liquid oils to find a suitable replacement. I wonder if this new way of processing will overcome the issue of trans fats.

Nutritionists are now revisiting unrefined tropical palm and coconut oils, which may not be as bad as once thought. These oils can tolerate high cooking temperatures and can offer numerous health benefits. I think this is a better alternative to trans fatty acids. Buy them in unrefined form.

American diets are currently overloaded with omega-6 and deficient in omega-3. The ratio in the current American diet is as high as 15:1. A healthier ratio would be 4:1 or even 2:1. However, for optimal health, your children need a balance between omega-3 and omega-6. Too much of one or the other can cause a variety of health problems.

For baked food and salads, unrefined olive oil is excellent but it should not be used for high temperature cooking. Healthier canola and sunflower oils that remain stable at high temperatures are coming onto the market. New seed oil crops are being bred to produce oils that don't need hydrogenation.

The healthy oils made with health (rather than shelf life) in mind are pressed from organically grown seeds and nuts, protected from destruction by light, air (oxygen), and heat during pressing, filtering, and found in dark opaque glass bottles.

If your children get the right kinds of fats from childhood, in the right amounts and balances, and prepare them using the right methods they build up their health. The wrong kinds of fats, the wrong amount or balances, or even the right kind of fats wrongly prepared can cause diseases of fatty degeneration.

GOLD NUGGETS

"The fact is your body needs fat. Fat plays a role in many of the complex biochemical processes that keep you alive, it helps you conserve precious body heat, and most important, it is your body's critical energy reserve. That's why Nature equipped you with some 35 million fat cells. But the trick is to get enough fat – and of the most healthy kinds – without getting too much." – Dr. Stuart Berger, author of *How to Be Your Own Nutritionist.*

"It is not only important to have the knowledge to avoid bad fats and oil and use good ones, but also know that industrial processing and frying can turn a good fat into a bad one, resulting in serious effects to your health." – Siegfried Gursche, the author of *Good Fats and Oil.*

"Most of the problems we blame on fats should actually be blamed on the destructive processing which fats have to undergo. Processing has nothing to do with health, but much to do with convenience, taste, shelf-life and profit. Processing removes most of the minerals, vitamins, protein, fiber, lecithin and antioxidants." – Dr. Udo Erasmus.

"Restaurants and fast food establishments used highly saturated lamb or beef tallow until the early 1980s, and it would be beneficial for everybody if they returned to that practice." – Mary G. Enig, PhD., another authority on fats.

"As for butter versus margarine, I trust cows more than chemists." – Joan Gussow.

Chapter 4

Take More Protein
from Plants

P rotein is made up of units called amino acids. There are 22 different amino acids in the food we eat, but our body can only make 13 of them from carbohydrates, fats, and other amino acids. The remaining nine are called essential amino acids as they cannot be produced by the body and must be obtained from your diet. From the nine essential amino acids, your body can make all of the rest of the non-essential amino acids and thus all the protein your body needs.

THE NEED FOR PROTEIN

Protein is one of the basic building blocks of your children's body, being about 16 percent of their total body weight. For instance their muscle, hair, skin, ligaments, and tendons are protein. Many of their hormones, DNA and thousands of enzymes are protein. Their disease-fighting immune system is nearly protein and it builds and repair body tissue cells.

Every one of their trillion cells is constantly aging, wearing out, and being replaced, hopefully by healthy cells. The lining of their digestive tract is replaced every six days, their skin is replaced every 28 days, and their bones are replaced every seven years.

The strength and health of the bones they will have in

seven years is right now being determined by the quality of protein they are currently consuming. Generous amounts of high quality protein are also needed to maintain rapid production of cells to support the immune system, prevent loss of lean muscle mass and boosting energy.

Unlike fats and glucose, your body has little capacity to store protein. If your children were to stop eating protein, their body would start to break down muscle for its needs within a day or so.

National Academy of Sciences recommends that 10 percent to 35 percent of daily calories should come from protein.

PROTEIN FROM ANIMAL SOURCES

Most recommendations for protein intake are based on animal-food sources such as meat, cow's milk and eggs. All are rich sources of saturated fats.

As far as possible, look for organic meat and poultry, and consume plenty of fish, especially cold water fish which are high in omega-3 fatty acids such as salmon, sardines, mackerel, trout and tuna.

Dairy products, besides been rich in saturated and cholesterol, may not be the best protein source since they create digestive problems for many people, such as excess gas, loose stools, mucous and congestion. Yeast infections and thrush also thrive on dairy foods.

PROTEIN FROM PLANT SOURCES

Studies show clearly that diets based solely on plant foods as sources of protein can be quite adequate to supply the recommended amounts of essential amino acids.

Encourage your children to eat protein from a variety of grains, vegetable and fruits, soy foods. Good proteins from plant sources include: Tofu or soymilk, nuts, avocados, sprouts, beans, lentils and legumes, besides having the added benefit of fiber, animal foods do not provide.

In order to stay in good health, an equal balance between animal proteins and vegetable proteins is better than eating more meat and less vegetables and fruits.

LIMIT EATING MEAT

There is a lot of controversy between vegetarians and meat eaters. Here are some reasons:

- Today, much of the red meat your children eat contains concentrated toxins such as pesticides, antibiotics, growth hormones and nitrates. These toxins when taken into their body are a potential danger to human health.

- Meat especially from farm reared animals contains 14 times as many pesticide residues as plant foods. It is estimated that fishes can accumulate up to nine million times the level of cancer-causing chemicals found in the waters in which they live.

- Meat and poultry contain quite a bit of fat, and about one-third of that fat is saturated. Saturated fatty acid in the diet increases Total cholesterol in the blood.

- Grilling, barbecuing, broiling, and pan-frying are more likely to produce heterocyclic amines (HCAs) which are carcinogenic chemicals. Heavy consumption of hot dogs, sausages and other processed meats could raise the risk of pancreatic cancer, according to the US Cancer Association.

If your children must eat meat, you can do the following:

- Feed them with organic, grass fed, beef, lamb, venison, bison, free range chicken and cold water fish caught in the wild, which will help them avoid residual pesticides, hormones, and antibiotics in conventionally raised animals.

- Minimize their consumption of grilled meats, which might be carcinogenic.

PUTTING IT TOGETHER

In America, we get a lot of quantity protein, but in my opinion, not enough quality protein is being met for optimal cellular health. I suggest you add a good quality protein drink to your children's usual diet which is a simple, healthy, and convenient way to assure optimal intake without the fat and cholesterol that is attached to meat, eggs, and many dairy products.

According to the Physicians Committee for Responsible Medicine, "To consume a diet that contains enough, but not too much, protein, simply replace animal products with grains, vegetables, legumes (peas, beans, and lentils), and fruits. As long as one is eating a variety of plant foods in sufficient quantity to maintain one's weight, the body gets plenty of protein."

GOLD NUGGETS

"Less than 70 years ago, more than 40 percent of the protein in the American diet came from grains, bread, and cereal. Currently, only 17 percent comes from these sources, along with another 15 percent from legumes, fruits, and vegetables, while two-thirds is from animal products. This trend, also noted in other industrialized Western countries, has been accompanied by a steady increase in heart disease and cancer deaths." – Charles Attwood, M.D.

"When you step back and look at the data, the optimum amount of red meat you eat should be zero." – Walter Willet, M.D.

"Did you ever see the customers in health-food stores? They are pale, skinny people who look half dead. In a steak house, you see robust, ruddy people. They're dying, of course, but they look terrific." – Bill Cosby.

"Condensed milk is wonderful. I don't see how they can get a cow to sit down on those little cans." – Fred Allen.

Chapter 5

Switch to Natural Sugars

S ugar is found everywhere. It is present naturally in fruits and vegetables, hidden in fruit-flavored drinks, energy bars, breakfast cereals, wholemeal bread, soups, crackers, mayonnaise, peanut butter, pickles, frozen pizza, canned fruits and vegetables, tomato juice, sugary snacks, sauces, salad dressings, preparations of meat and other products, just to name a few.

Many of these sugary foods are found in grocery shelves, vending machines, pubs, restaurants and school menus. This makes it difficult for your children to avoid them; unless you are preparing their food from scratch.

WORRYING TRENDS

Today, our children's food has twice the amount of refined sugar in them, as compared to 30 years ago. A typical child's breakfast today looks probably like this: Processed breakfast cereal (sugar) with milk (more sugar), toast and jam (even more sugar), served with a glass of fruit juice from concentrates (still more sugar).

Follow the wise advice of Dr. Leo Galland, a writer of children's health, "My first line of advice to parents is to keep their children away from sugary cereals, pancakes or waffles with syrup, soft drinks, candy, cakes, cookies, doughnuts, ice cream, frozen yogurt and chocolate. Every ounce of reduction helps. Sugar alone does not cause hyperactivity, but it does reduce the nutritional quality of the diet and may aggravate other food intolerances."

This is a worrying trend for all parents. As parents, begin to educate your children early about sugar, if you want to bring up healthy disease free kids.

THE NEED FOR SUGAR

Adding sugar to food enhances taste, but has the negative effect of boosting calories. Sugar flavors really help make eating pleasurable.

Sugar acts as a bulking agent (ice cream, baked goods) and as a preservative (jams, fruits), and add sweetness to beverages and carbonated drinks. Sugar contributes significantly to the flavor, aroma, texture, color and body of a variety of foods. Sugar syrups protect frozen and canned fruits from browning and withering.

It is possible that the earlier you expose an infant to "sweet", the more likely they will crave for it as they grow up.

The goal should be to eat as little sugar as possible. Sugars from fruits are acceptable, but any sugar from processed foods should be minimized. Granted, that's hard to do, but just try to keep it as low as possible. Sugar has no nutritional benefit.

A bowl of sweetened cereal for breakfast, a cup of fruit yogurt for a snack, and a scoop of sherbet for dessert: You've just had more than 20 teaspoons of sugar without opening the sugar jar.

Today, Americans on an average are taking 22 teaspoons of added sugar along with their food daily. Most of the sugar eaten comes from sucrose or table sugar and high fructose corn syrup. Much of the increase is due to the consumption of soft drinks.

Nutrition experts agree that too much sugar is unhealthy. Unfortunately, they could not agree on how much is too much. It is difficult to avoid sugar as they are hidden in all processed foods.

The best advice I can give is to eat foods that are close to nature and don't add sugar at the table or in your children's drink or when you are cooking. If this is not possible, go for the natural sugars but still in moderation.

TYPES OF SUGAR

There are many types of sugars: Natural sugar, refined sugar, artificial sweeteners and sugar substitute. Each type differs from one another by its use, sweetness, flavor, caloric and nutritional values.

Natural Sugar

The following is a list of natural sugar that is not processed, contain fewer calories and contain more nutrients than other sugars. Natural sugar is considered to produce less of a shock to the body's blood sugar level.

Although no sugar is without problems, natural sugars seem to have less negative impact upon the body. Natural sugar is not an enemy per se. It has undeniable nutritional benefits as long as it not refined, not eaten alone and taken in moderation. A word of caution: If you child is a diabetic you need to monitor their body's response to natural sugars.

The natural sugars include:

Fructose

Fructose is often referred to as fruit sugar because of its presence in fruits. It is one and a half times sweeter than sucrose. The sugars in fruit are balanced with vitamins and fiber to slow the glucose absorption; making for longer lasting energy foods with far greater nutritional value than sucrose.

It is considered a nutritive sweetener unlike refined

sugar (sucrose) that contains only empty calories. Fructose sugar is sweeter than table sugar but it does not produce the roller coaster effect of your blood sugar.

It turns "ugly" when it is commercially refined from corn, sugar beets, and sugar cane. Since it is about 70 percent sweeter than sucrose, many food manufacturers now use refined fructose to replace sucrose in canned and frozen fruit, soft drinks, juices, and a great many other packaged foods.

Honey

Raw, unpasteurized honey can be considered a great substitute for refined sugar. The highest quality honey is not processed, not filtered, nor refined. However, use it in moderation. Never give raw honey to children younger than 2 years old because of the risk of infant botulism.

On average, honey is nearly 20 percent water, and contains about 40 percent fructose, 30 percent glucose and 1 percent sucrose. The remainder is a mixture of other sugars and minute traces of naturally occurring acids, vitamins, minerals and enzymes.

Maltose

It is a form of sugar resulting from "malting" certain grains together with natural enzymes. Two of the most popular forms are barley malt and brown rice syrup. Maltose is about one-third as sweet as sucrose.

Glucose

Glucose is in nearly all plant foods. It is about two-third as sweet as sucrose. Glucose is also the form that all sugars are broken down to by your bodies to be utilized for energy production.

Also known as dextrose, glucose is found naturally in fruit, honey, and corn. Glucose turns unhealthy when is produced commercially by hydrolyzing (splitting) corn starch.

Lactose
Lactose is naturally present sugar in milk. So you cannot skip this sugar if you are drinking milk.

Pure Maple Syrup
Pure maple syrup is unrefined syrup made from the sap of the maple tree, unlike refined maple sugar which contains a high percentage of sucrose. Forty liters of maple sap is required to produce one liter of pure maple syrup. It is a highly concentrated natural sugar with a delicate flavor and a mild taste. Because of its high sweetening power, use it in small quantities.

Pure maple syrup is high in zinc, calcium, magnesium, manganese and some B vitamins. The maple flavored syrup sold in supermarkets are usually corn syrups (refined sugar) consisting of 20 percent maple syrup sugar with artificial colorings and flavorings added.

Pure maple syrup can be used over pancakes or waffles, as a sauce over ice cream or puddings, and even in many elaborate "gourmet" recipes.

Agave Syrup

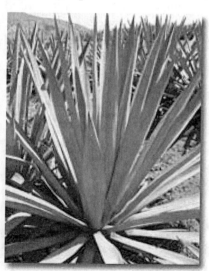

Agave is a sweetener extracted from the fruit of the Mexican cactus, and traditionally used to make tequila. The sap or juice contains 90 percent fructose.

Agave syrup is not as sweet or thick as honey and can be used as a honey substitute. Choose raw agave that is closer to its natural state than one processed at higher temperatures. The dark raw agaves have lower glycemic index than the lighter version.

Agave is rich in vitamin B, C, D, E, calcium, iron, phosphorus, magnesium, potassium, zinc, selenium, and chromium.

Agave nectar is a wonderful sweetener for beverages, cereals, salad dressing and BBQ sauce.

Sucanat

It's an organic sweetener made from 100 percent certified organic sugar cane. Unlike refined and processed white sugar, sucanat retains its molasses content. The juice is extracted by a mechanical process, heated and cooled at which point the small brown grainy crystals are formed.

This can be used as a good alternative to commercially produced sweeteners, refined white and brown sugar. Sucanat is about the closest thing you can get to pure sugar cane, right from the plant.

Sucanat ranks the highest in nutritional value. Besides containing a smaller proportion of sucrose, it also contains vitamins, minerals, and trace elements and carbohydrate – all of which refined sugar does not have.

Amasake

Amasake is a creamy, rich, sweetener made from fermented rice. This process is similar to the creation of rice wine, or sake. This sweetener can be used as a replacement for evaporated cane sugar or even honey.

It contains all of the nutritional benefits of whole grain brown rice, including fiber, enzymes that aids in digestion, cellulose, and most of the essential amino acids.

Stevia (Stevia Rebaudiana)
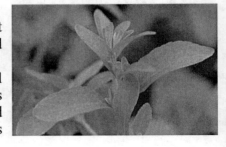
Stevia is known as a "sweet herb" by natives of South and Central America for centuries.

It is an all-natural herbal sweetener that contains no chemicals, no calories and no effect on blood sugar. It's

200 times sweeter than refined sugar.

Refined Sugars

Every day we're hearing more and more about the dangers of refined sugar and how it affects your child's health. So what are refined sugars? Refined sugars are processed sugar from plant sources that have their natural fibers, vitamins, amino acid and minerals stripped off. Not only does it totally lack nutrients, but refined sugar actually robs your body of vitamins, minerals and enzymes.

Here is a list showing the most common refined sugar you often come across in your grocery counter. Refined sugars are carbohydrates as they come from plants.

Sucrose

Sucrose is commonly known as table sugar or the white crystalline sugar you put in your coffee. It is also the most common sugar for household and industrial use. It's equivalent to refined white oils.

They are refined from cane or beet juice with all its vitamins, minerals, protein, fiber and water stripped off. Sucrose is empty calories and has the worse negative effects on your body when compared to other types of sugars. Sucrose provides four calories per gram (approximately 16 calories per teaspoon).

Sucrose is America's number one food additive to enhance the flavor of foods before high fructose corn syrup came to the scene. Believe it or not, Americans consume more sucrose than all the other 2,600 or so food additives put together. This doesn't even take into account the obvious sugary products found in processed foods like candies, cakes, ice cream, cookies, doughnuts, and soda pop. The one exception is salt, but it ranks a very distant second.

Light Molasses

Light molasses is the syrup remaining after the first extraction of sugar from sugar cane. It is often used as syrup for pancakes and waffles or stirred into hot cereals such as oatmeal. It is 65 percent sucrose.

Brown Sugar (Light and Dark)
It is refined cane or beet sugar with molasses still on the sugar crystals. Most U.S. sugar manufacturers refine the sugar completely and then add the molasses back in specific amounts. Most of the brown sugar sold in supermarkets is simply refined sugar with molasses added.

One tablespoon of brown sugar has 48 calories against 45 calories for white sugar. It has 96 percent sucrose.

The rich, full flavor of dark brown sugar makes it good for gingerbread, mincemeat, baked beans, and other full flavored food.

Maple Sugar
It contains 65 percent sucrose. Maple sugar is dehydrated maple syrup. It is twice as sweet as white sugar. Maple sugar candy is so sweet, only a small amount can be eaten at a time.

High Fructose Corn Syrup (HFCS)
HFCS is different from the healthy fructose found in fresh fruits. High fructose corn syrup (HFCS) has replaced sucrose in most American prepared foods as the most popular sweetener.

This sugar must be avoided as much as possible as research shows it can cause obesity and high blood pressure. (Dr. Richard Johnson of the University of Denver Colorado)

It is made by using acids and enzymes to break down the corn syrup. HFCS contains 14 percent of fructose with a glycemic index of 89, which is only slightly less than that of table sugar, at 92. In contrast, natural fructose has a glycemic index of 32.

HFCS are used in many of today's baked goods, sauces, jellies, salad dressings, powdered drink mixes, fruit drinks and juices, and frozen desserts like pudding and ice milk.

Downside of Refined Sugars

Nancy Appelton, a well known researcher and author, has given 146 reasons why sugar can harm the body. If you want the full list, read her book entitled, "Lick the sugar habit."

"Sugar contributes empty carbohydrate calories, which Americans certainly don't need. We are ingesting too many calories in general. Our high intake of sugars and refined starches increase the risk of diabetes and heart disease, even after accounting for their effects on weight," says Walter Willett, M.D., chair of the Department of Nutrition at the Harvard School of Public Health.

Some nutritionist is now naming sugar as the "new fat." Eating sugar may be as bad as eating saturated fats as any excessive intake of any type of sugar will be converted by the body into triglycerides or body fat. If sugar is taken consistently over a prolonged period of time, it can harm the health of your children in the foreseeable future.

It also suppress the immune system and upsets the body's mineral balance.

Refined sugars also have a very powerful shock effect, especially in children, leaving them hyperactive, tired and loss of concentration.

Excessive weight gain from refines sugars can lead to obesity. According to the American Heart Association, obesity is an independent risk factor for cardiovascular disease because it adversely affects cholesterol and triglyceride levels, blood pressure and blood glucose levels.

Added sugars have virtually no nutritional value. They're no substitute for whole foods which are rich in vitamins and nutrients.

Artificial Sweeteners (Non Nutritive)

Many people have turned to artificial sweeteners to satisfy their cravings for sweet. Because they are much sweeter than sugar, it takes a tiny amount to create the same sweetness. Artificial sweeteners are low in calories.

Artificial sweeteners are organic compound that do not

contain carbohydrates, so they do not cause blood sugar to elevate. They are useful in diabetes management when used properly.

They are "tooth-friendly." They do not cause tooth decay like sucrose does. The following artificial sweeteners are commonly used as table-top sweeteners and approved by the Federal Drug Administration:

Aspartame (Equal and NutraSweet)

Aspartame is 200 times sweeter than sucrose. It has about 4 calories per gram, but because of its intense sweetness, very little is used at any one time. It dominates the packaged food, soft drink and table top sweetener market. Because it is not generally heat stable, it is not used for cooking.

It is so easy to overdose on this sweetener because Aspartame is found in so many products. So if you want to minimize taking Aspartame, learn to read labels.

Side effects: Headaches, seizures, and mood swings. People with a rare condition called phenylketonuria (PKU) should not take Aspartame.

Acesulfame K (Sweet One or Sunnette)

It is 200 times sweeter than table sugar and sold in packets or tablets.

It is also found in some baked goods, frozen desserts, candies, beverages, cough drops, and breath mints. Unfortunately, Acesulfame K is considered to be a potential carcinogen.

Sucralose (Splenda)

It tastes like sugar, but is 600 times sweeter than sugar. Food manufacturers value sucralose because it is the most heat stable of all the artificial sweeteners.

The claim that Sucralose is made of sugar is misleading. It is made through a chemical process by adding chlorine atoms to sucrose. There is not been enough studies to prove that it is safe. Some research shows it is detrimental to health.

Saccharin (Sweet 'N'Low, Sweet Twin and Necta Sweet)
Saccharin is 300 times sweeter than table sugar. This sweetener is sold in liquid, tablets, packets, and in bulk.

Saccharin has a warning on its label: *"Use of this product may be hazardous to your health. This product contains saccharin, which has been determined to cause cancer in laboratory animals."*

In spite of this warning, this sweetener continues to be widely used as a low-caloric sweetener. Saccharin is one artificial sweetener that is widely used in pharmaceuticals, vitamins, cosmetics products, as well as in baked and processed foods.

The Downside of Artificial Sweeteners
They are non-nutritive. They may aid diabetics but they have been linked to medical problems such as cancer, migraines, depression, birth defects, seizures, behavior changes, anemia, sexual and thyroid dysfunction and more.

The biggest drawback to this class of sweeteners is that, they all involve the use of artificial chemicals. They are all hidden in the processed foods, bottled and package drinks, so to know their existence you need to read labels.

Artificial sweeteners aren't any better than HFCS. Studies have found that rats ate more after consuming an artificially sweetened drink than they did after sipping water containing sucrose.

Sugar Alcohol (Nutritive)
Sugar alcohols are a type of carbohydrate. Their structure resembles that of sugar and alcohol. They are not as sweet as sucrose or artificial sweeteners.

Often foods containing sugar alcohols are labeled "sugar-free." Sugar alcohols have been found to be a beneficial substitute for refined sugar as it reduces fluctuation in blood sugar, prevent dental cavities, and lowers caloric intake.

Sugar alcohols occur naturally in a wide variety of fruits and vegetables, but are commercially produced from other carbohydrates such as sucrose, glucose, and starch.

As a sugar substitute, they provide only 2.4 kilocalories per gram compared to 4 grams for sucrose. According to the American Dietetic Association excess consumption of sugar alcohol can lead to abdominal gas, diarrhea and weight gain.

Food products labeled "sugar-free," include hard candies, cookies, chewing gums, soft drinks and throat lozenges. They are frequently used in toothpaste and mouthwash.

Xylitol

It is natural sweetener produced from the fibers of fruits and vegetables. Pure xylitol is a white, crystalline, natural substance that looks and tastes like sugar. Its sweetness is equal to sugar, but it contains 40 percent fewer calories.

It reduces tooth decay, has been endorsed by dental associations and is used extensively in sugar-free products such as chewing gums, hard candies, diet foods and toothpaste.

Unlike many artificial sweeteners, it leaves no unpleasant aftertaste. Xylitol has no known toxic levels but taken in excess of 90 gm/day may have a laxative effect.

Mannitol

It occurs naturally in pineapples, olives, asparagus, sweet potatoes and carrots. Mannitol is extracted from seaweed. It has approximately 90 percent of the sweetness of sucrose but it has just half the calories.

They are found in chocolates, hard candies, baked goods, confections, ice cream and chewing gum.

Sorbitol

Found naturally in fruits and vegetables. It is manufactured from corn syrup and has only 50 percent of the relative sweetness of sugar. It has less of a tendency to cause diarrhea compared to Mannitol. It is often found in sugar-free gums and candies.

Lactitol

It has about 30-40 percent of sugar's sweetening power. They are found in food products such as ice cream, chocolate, hard and soft candies, baked goods, sugar-reduced preserves and chewing gums.

Isomalt

It is 45-65 percent as sweet as sugar and does not tend to lose its sweetness or break down during the heating process. It is often used in hard candies, toffee, cough drops and lollipops.

The Downside of Sugar Alcohol

High intake of foods containing sugar alcohols can lead to abdominal gas and diarrhea because they are not completely absorbed in your body.

The presence of sugar alcohols in foods does not mean that you can eat unlimited quantities. Sugar alcohols are lower in calories, gram for gram, than sugar. They are not calorie-free, and if eaten in large enough quantities, the calories can be comparable to sugar-containing foods.

Weight gain has been seen when these products are overeaten. The American Diabetes Association claims that sugar alcohols are acceptable if taken moderately.

REDUCE SUGAR INTAKE

Having identified the good and dark side of different types of sugars available to your children, let us now work out some ways to cut back on sugar. Getting sugar completely out your children's diet isn't easy, but lessening their intake is.

Your challenge is to begin by making small changes in your children's liking for refined sugar as most children's products are loaded with added sugars. So next time you go shopping, teach your children how to read food labels to identify the type of sugar the food contains.

Like fats, sugar has its good and ugly side. As sugar

goes by more than fifty names, you need to learn to differentiate the good from the unhealthy ones and guide your children to take in moderation the ones that do less damage to their body.

Here are some great ways you can take, to slowly decrease sugar in your children's diet:

- Become more aware of where sugar shows up in their food. Start reading labels for hidden sugars in foods. Here are some terms on food labels that indicate the presence of refined sugars in a product: White sugar, brown sugar, icing sugar, invert sugar, corn syrup, high fructose corn syrup, maple syrup, honey, molasses, brown rice syrup, cane juice, evaporated cane juice, all fruit concentrates, and all words ending in "ose" such as dextrose, fructose, lactose, glucose, maltose and sucrose.

- Make a goal to stay under 40 grams (10 teaspoons) of sugar per day. A major portion must come from natural sugars. Involve your kids in counting and tallying them.

- Lower the sugar on foods your kids love. For example, if they love cereals or peanut butter, buy the product with the lowest sugar content.

- Limit TV and commercials that encourage sugary snacks.

- Set an example. Don't consume sugary food in front of your children or stock up sugary foods in your pantry.

- Do not add sugar to your children's coffee, tea or cereals or any food. Your children are already daily taking sugars that are hidden in most of their food.

- Avoid all canned and bottled sodas, powdered drinks, sports drinks, and fruit juices; instead encourage them to drink plenty of purified clean water until it becomes habitual. They all contain artificial sweeteners.

- Exercise is a great antidote for sugar cravings. That's because when you exercise, your body breaks down glycogen and releases glucose molecules into your bloodstream, effectively giving you a sugar boost.

- Load up their snacks or part of their meals with vegetables and legumes such as beans, peas, and lentils. These foods are loaded with fiber and nutrients. Fiber gives a nice, long, steady release of sugar into the bloodstream, reducing hunger pangs. This will help your children to cut back on their sugar intake.

- Don't be afraid to omit the sugar in salads, dressings, casseroles, or soups.

- Ration rather than ban. It is better to ration the amount of sugar they consume.

- Instead of adding sugar to your cooking, add spices and unrefined salt to bring up the flavor in your food.

IN A NUTSHELL

The goal should be to eat as little sugar as possible, but if they do, as much as possible must come from natural sugar such as stevia, sucanat or agave syrup. It is vital to reduce your children's intake of artificial sweeteners, sugar alcohol, table sugar or refined sugar hidden in processed foods, as consistent and prolonged intake is hazardous to their health.

GOLD NUGGETS

"The solution to sugar cravings is first to understand what our basic nutritional needs are and how to adapt them into our lifestyle, so we can enjoy natural sweet treats without developing the addictive feeling that requires a sweet after a meal." – Verne Varona, author of *Nature's Cancer Fighting Foods*.

"Research shows that right after you eat a high sugar meal, the function of the cells in your immune system drops dramatically." – Dr. Christine Horner, author of *Walking the Warrior Goddess*.

"The bottom line is that sugar upsets the body chemistry and suppresses the immune system. Once the immune system becomes suppressed, the door is opened to infectious and degenerative diseases. The stronger the immune system the easier it is for the body to fight infectious and degenerative diseases." – Nancy Appleton, Ph.D.

Chapter 6

Throw Away the Salt Shaker

A s salt plays a vital role in your children's health, I am going to devote a whole chapter to help you, as parents, to have a deeper understanding of the nature of salt, how different types of salt work in the body and the health issues involved. The knowledge gained can guide you to select the salt that promotes the health of your children from young.

ALL SALTS ARE NOT CREATED EQUAL

Salt is not purely sodium, as salt is made up of 40 percent sodium and 60 percent chloride, while sodium is just sodium.

Salt is commonly used as preservatives, emulsifiers, stabilizers, buffers or acid regulator, neutralizers, flavor enhancers, color fixative in cured meat, chelating agent, thickeners, bleaching agent, and as anti-caking agents.

Salt can be sourced from the sea (sea salt) or from mineral deposits (rock salt). Sea salt is made by evaporating sea water while rock salt is mined from deposits that were left behind by seas or oceans that had dried up.

Today, between 65 and 85 percent of the salt we eat, comes from salt hidden in processed food and beverages and not in what you add to your cooking or at the dinner table. In fact, it is safe to say your children don't need to add salt to their food or drink.

When buying salt, it is important to find out where the salt comes from, how it was harvested, whether it is refined or unrefined, its quality and flavor.

In today's market, we now have two distinct choices when it comes to salt: Sea salt (unrefined) or table salt (refined).

Sea Salt (Unrefined)

Unrefined salt usually comes from seawater, but in some cases it can be obtained from rock salt.

Sea Salt is naturally harvested by channeling sea or ocean water into man-made pools; along protected shoreline. The sunlight, along with some wind, will evaporate the water and turn it into sea salt. The salt is then dissolved in water and the impurities removed by evaporation.

Your children's intake of salt should mainly come from unrefined sea salt. Unrefined salt is beneficial to the human body because our blood has the same chemical balance of sodium, potassium and calcium found in salt from the ocean.

Sea salt (unrefined) is 98 percent sodium chloride and 2 percent trace minerals such as iron, magnesium, calcium, potassium, vanadium, bromine, silicon, phosphorus and sulfur but a poor source of iodine. Unrefined sea salt does not contain added sugar, anti-caking ingredients or potassium or iodine. It is this property that makes unrefined sea salt, a healthy option.

Unrefined sea salt has a strong flavor. Salt is available in fine or coarse grain. Unrefined salt tends to be off-white, gray, pink or a mix of colors because of the presence of trace minerals.

Main sources of sea salt come from the Mediterranean Sea, the North Sea, and the Atlantic Ocean.

Here are three popular unrefined quality salts you might want to consider to replace your salt shaker:

Fleur de Sel (Flower of Salt)

Is a fine quality French salt produced only in the towns of Guerande, along the coast of Brittany in France. It has been referred to as "the caviar of salt" by food aficionados around the globe.

It is hand harvested, unprocessed, unrefined, and unadulterated. Due to the small size of the crystals, *fleur de sel* dissolves faster than regular salt. It is often slightly grey due to the sandy minerals collected in the process of harvesting. It has a high concentration of minerals such as calcium, magnesium and iron.

It is used to finish a dish. It is a natural compliment to fresh raw vegetables and salads and can elevate the flavor of grilled meats and fish.

Due to its relative scarcity, Fleur de Sel is one of the more expensive salts. The most famous of these salts is *Fleur de Sel de Guérande.*

Himalayan Salt

Is 100 percent natural, unrefined and unpolluted pink, translucent crystals. It is harvested from the foothills of the Himalayas. This marine fossil salt comes from the ancient sea with rich minerals such as calcium, magnesium, potassium, copper and iron.

Celtic Sea Salt

Is another good alternative to refined seas salt. The main trace minerals found in Celtic sea salt are iodine, iron, calcium, magnesium, manganese, potassium and zinc with no chemical and preservatives nor any other additives.

It is hand harvested using the Celtic method of wooden rakes allowing no metal to touch the salt. Celtic salts are available in coarse, stone ground fine and extra fine grain and it is light grey in color.

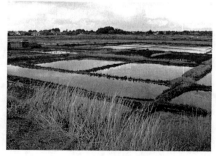

Celtic Salt imparts a pure, fresh taste to your meals, rather than the harsh flavor of table salt. Use Celtic salt for all flavoring just as you would in place of table salt.

Table Salt (Refined Salt)
Table salt is the most common kind of salt found in most kitchens. It is made from the terrestrial salt deposits which are mined, heat-blasted then chemically treated (iodized, bleached and diluted with chemical anti-caking agents). This refining process literally removes the valuable trace minerals present in the salt, other than sodium and chloride. When it comes to health, the sodium content is what we are concerned about.

Refined salt is 97.5 percent sodium chloride and approximately 2.5 percent chemical additives. Table salt is a fine-grained salt which makes it easy to dissolve in water. Because of its fine grain, a single teaspoon of table salt contains more salt than a tablespoon of unrefined sea salt.

Refined salt or sodium is full of chemical additives that are harmful to health. Common sodium additives found in processed foods include: Disodium guanylate (flavor enhancer), sodium alginate (thickener), sodium benzoate (preservative), sodium bicarbonate (texture enhancer), monosodium glutamate (also called MSG), sodium nitrite/nitrate (curing meats and sausages) and many more.

Sources of Refined Salt
The main source of salt in the diet comes from processed foods, naturally occurring at the table and during cooking. See diagram below.

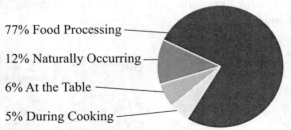

77% Food Processing
12% Naturally Occurring
6% At the Table
5% During Cooking

Source: Mattes RD, Donnelly D. Relative contributions of dietary sodium sources. *Journal of American College of Nutrition*

Highly Processed Foods
Processed foods are thought to account for around 77 percent of the average person's salt intake. Salt is added to processed foods to aid preservation and to improve taste.

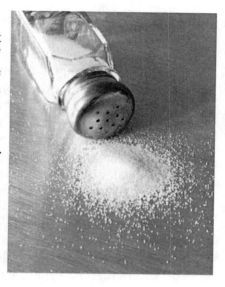

Some examples of processed foods containing sodium addictives are: Meats (bacon, sausage, and ham, tuna, corned beef), canned soups and vegetables, bread, breakfast cereals, cheese, salad dressing, sauces of all kinds, packaged or frozen items, prepared take-home dishes, instant foods, and most meals eaten at restaurants or fast foods. The list is endless.

Naturally Occurring
Sodium are found naturally in seafood such as fish, prawns, crabs, lobsters, and seaweed, in plant foods such as celery, carrots, cauliflower, pineapples, jackfruits and in eggs nuts.

At the Table
Do not add refined salt or the salt shaker to your food at the table. You are already taking enough sodium from sodium hidden in processed foods.

During Cooking
Reduce adding salt to your daily cooking. Instead use herbs to add flavor to your food.

THE VALUE OF SALT

Salt is an essential nutrient. The body may endure periods of lack of food, but without salt and water, the living cells of your body would quickly perish.

Your body contains about eight ounces of salt. The amount of salt is regulated in your bodies by our kidneys and by perspiration. It is the excessive consumption of refined salt (sodium addictives) found in processed food mentioned earlier that is unfavorable to your child's health.

Sodium is an electrolyte. Electrolytes main task is to carry nutrients in and out of your body cells and waste products and excess water out of the cells. Assist the kidneys to remove excess acidity from the cells in the body.

They carry messages along your nerves, help control your heartbeat, regulate blood pressure and blood volume and help maintain proper acidity or pH of the blood.

Salt is needed from blood sugar regulation to bone density to circulatory health, contraction and relaxation of the body's muscles.

Deficiency in salt can cause heart palpitations, dehydration, low blood pressure, muscle cramps, and low libido.

DANGERS OF EXCESS SALT INTAKE

Salt per se is not harmful to health but it is when we take in the wrong kind of salt and in excessive amount that it becomes harmful. Just as there are different kinds of sugar and fats, there are also different kinds of salt.

Most of the health issues caused by salt should be blamed on the commercial processing methods which turn good salt that "heals" to one that "kills." The typical modern refined salt products can be compared to refined sugar, refined flour and refined oils and fats that have their nutrients stripped by commercial processing.

The American Medical Association is so serious about the health hazards of sodium that it has called on the Food and Drug Administration (FDA) to revoke the status of salt as a "generally recognized as safe" and to set limits to the amount of salt that can be added to highly processed foods and those served in restaurants. The Association also called on food manufacturers and restaurants to gradually cut the sodium in their foods over the next 10 years to achieve a minimum of a 50 percent sodium reduction.

Nutrition researchers are still trying to trace the role sodium plays in hypertension. Not all scientist, agree that salt intake is linked to high blood pressure. New research is linking the cause to imbalance between sodium and potassium in the blood.

HOW MUCH SALT DO YOUR CHILDREN NEED?

Whether you use sea salt, table salt or some other type of salt, below is a rough guide on the amount of salt babies and children require daily:

- No more than 1 gram per day from 0-12 months
- 2 grams (0.8 gram sodium) per day from 1-3 years
- 3 grams (1.2 gram sodium) per day from 4-6 years
- 5 grams (2 gram sodium) per day from 7-10 years
- 6 grams (2.4 gram sodium) a day from 11 years onwards

One gram of salt contains about 400 mg of sodium. One teaspoon of salt is equivalent to about 2,400 milligrams of sodium. Use the teaspoon method to keep track of your children's daily sodium intake preferably from unrefined sea salt.

Babies and children only need a very small amount of salt in their diet. However, because salt is "hidden" in many ready-made foods, such as bread, baked beans and even cookies, it can be easy to have too much.

FDA GUIDELINES ON SODIUM LABELS

The following is a guide to the phrases used in sodium labeling as defined by the FDA:

Sodium Free: Less than 5 mg sodium per serving

Very Low Sodium: Less than 35 mg sodium per serving

Low Sodium: Less than 140 mg sodium per serving

Reduced Sodium: 75 percent reduction in sodium content from original product

Unsalted: Processed without salt

HOW TO REDUCE SALT INTAKE?

To reduce salt, the key is to cut back gradually on the amount of salt you use. Your taste buds will adjust to less salt. Here are a couple of ways you can help reduce salt in your children's food:

•   Educate your children about the dangers of eating more salt than the body requires. Scientific evidence suggests that dietary habits in childhood influence eating patterns in later life.

•   Stop adding table salt to food once it is served.

•   Don't add salt to your cooking. Taste your food before you salt it; it may not need more salt. Instead use fresh garlic or garlic powder, ginger, hot peppers, browned onions, lemon or lime juice, flavored vinegar, cumin, nutmeg, cinnamon, fresh ground pepper, tarragon, oregano, onion, mint, chives, parsley and many others as an alternative to salt when cooking.

- Cut down on salty snacks – choose unsalted versions of nuts, snack on dried fruits, fruits and vegetables.

- Cut down on heavily salted foods such as bacon, cheese, ready-prepared meals.

- Choose fresh, frozen or canned food items without added salts.

- Food products that are seasoned, barbecued, blackened, breaded, smoked, pickled, marinated, all contain high amount of sodium.

- Watch for hidden sodium overload in restaurant foods. Specify what you want and how you want it prepared when dining out. Ask for your dish to be prepared without salt.

- Curb condiments: Ketchup, mustard, relish, tartar sauce, pickles and similar add-ons are loaded with salt. Use sliced fresh tomatoes, pepper and herbs instead.

- Keep takeaways and fast foods such as burgers, fried chicken and pizza as an occasional treat.

- If you think your meals are high in sodium, balance them by adding high-potassium foods, such as fresh fruits, vegetables and nuts.

- Sodium comes in many forms, not just as table salt, or sodium chloride. There's also sodium benzoate (a preservative), sodium nitrate (found in processed meats), monosodium glutamate (the flavor enhancer known as MSG), as well as sodium in baking powder and baking soda. All add to your total daily sodium intake.

- The words "soda" (referring to sodium bicarbonate, or baking soda) and "sodium" and the symbol "Na" on food products indicate the presence of sodium compounds.

- Several major food companies, in an effort to lower sodium content in their packaged foods, have experimented with the use of potassium chloride by adding bitter blockers and masking agents.

- Food labels often state the sodium, rather than the salt content of food. To calculate the amount of salt in a product, multiply the sodium content by two-and-a-half times.

BOTTOM LINE

Salt is not the enemy, and by no means should it be eliminated from your child's diet. In fact, you need salt to survive. No food supplementation can equal the wealth of minerals found in unrefined sea salt. What you need to do is to replace table salt with natural sea salt. However, still take unrefined salt in moderation.

Salt substitutes are available, but they are not for everyone. Some replace the sodium with potassium and can be harmful to people with a medical condition. Talk to your doctor before using salt substitutes.

Wherever possible season your foods with herbs and spices. Grill, bake, broil, boil, steam or roast your food as much as possible.

GOLD NUGGETS

"If by eating less salt, the world's population reduced its average blood pressure by a single millimeter of mercury, would prevent several hundred thousand deaths a year. That would do more for worldwide deaths than the abolition of cancer." – Richard Peto, epidemiologist, Oxford University

"If you wanted to design a diet for children guaranteed to lead to strokes and heart attacks in later life, it would closely resemble the high salt, high fat diet that many children eat now." – Professor Graham MacGregor, professor of Cardiovascular Medicine at George's Hospital, London

Chapter 7

Make Purified Water
the Drink of Choice

Water is often the forgotten nutrient. Next to air, water is the second most important element required by any living being. It is absolutely necessary for growing children to drink enough clean water. However, how much water your children need daily depends on how much they sweat during exercise, the climate and their weight and general health.

You can actually survive without food for months, but without water you would not survive for long. Fortunately, the body has a built-in mechanism to warn you when you need to replace the water you lose daily from breathing, perspiration, bowel movement and urination. It is called thirst!

DAILY NEED OF WATER

It is generally recommended that children consume at least six to eight glasses of water daily (1.5 to 2 liter). However, the Institute of Medicine of the National Academies, Washington DC (2004), recommends that children above 14 ought to have an average fluid intake of about 11 glasses daily (about 2.6 liter).

A recent survey reveals that most children and adults fall short of drinking eight glasses of water a day. Only 34 percent actually drink this amount, while 10 percent said they do not drink water at all. However, most Americans including children instead drink an average of nearly six servings a day of caffeinated beverages such as coffee, soda and other carbonated and fizzy drinks, causing the body to lose more water.

THE HEALTH BENEFITS OF WATER

Water makes up approximately 60 percent of the body weight. Your body is over 75 percent water in one form or another. Every system in the body depends on water. Lack of water can lead to dehydration, a condition that occurs when you don't have enough water to carry out normal body functions. Children can be taught to recognize symptoms of mild dehydration by the color of their urine: Deep yellow in color, smelly and cloudy.

The brain is about 75 percent water. Poor hydration can affect a child's mental performance and learning ability. A loss of three percent of total body water will cause fatigue and 10 percent is seriously life threatening. Even mild dehydration may cause tiredness, reduced alertness and ability to concentrate.

Continuous long term dehydration can increase the risk of a number of health problems: Constipation, continence problems, kidney and urinary tract infections, kidney stones, and some cancers. The key is to keep well hydrated throughout the day with water as opposed to any other fluids or other beverages.

Water assists in digestion, transports nutrients, enzymes and proteins into cells while removing waste and toxins from the body. It also, aids the lungs, heart and blood vessels, helps metabolize fat, keep the body to stay cool and energizes the brain and body.

Iranian medical doctor F. Batmanghelidj, author of *Your Body's Many Cries for Water*, says that he does not count coffee, tea, sodas and juices toward your daily allotment of water. In fact, he states that caffeine is a diuretic and should be avoided. Children who drink lots of tea, coffee, hot chocolate and carbonated drinks tend to have tired-looking, greasy skin and spots.

Water can decrease your appetite. When you drink water, your stomach gets full and your appetite decreases.

Drinking water burns extra calories. Drinking 18 ounces of water increases your metabolic rate by about 30 percent for about 40 minutes.

It is important to teach children good water drinking habit. Get your children into the habit of carrying a water bottle with purified water wherever they go. This will help them to avoid drinking soft drinks and carbonated beverages. When using reusable water bottles, drain, rinse and clean the bottle before filling them with drinking water.

The key is to keep well hydrated throughout the day with pure clean water; as opposed to any other fluids or other beverages.

BEYOND THE TAP

There are more than 60,000 different chemicals on the market today. In one way or another, many of these chemicals find their way into your water. Today, your children may be drinking the residues from fertilizers, pesticides, herbicides, and industrial wastes, fluoride, chlorine, dioxins and much more which are detrimental to adult and children's health. Therefore it's critically important that we take steps to protect yourselves and your families with a clean source of water.

Here are some good sources of water beyond your tap water:

Reverse Osmosis Water
Reverse osmosis filtration is a water treatment process in which tap water is purified by forcing pressurized water through a very fine membrane.

Reverse osmosis is a good choice if you're concerned about a wide range of contaminants: Lead, copper, arsenic, cadmium, chlorine, chromium, mercury, pesticides, salt, sulfates, cysts, and nitrates.

It can improve the taste of water for people who do not like the taste of dissolved mineral solids.

Its main disadvantage is that it wastes two to four gallons of tap water for every gallon that gets filtered. The less rejected water it generates, the shorter the life span of the membrane, as rejected water helps keep the membrane clean.

Reverse osmosis treatment systems remove vital minerals like calcium and magnesium from drinking water.

A flaw or tear to the membrane could allow untreated water to flow through the unit without removing disease-causing organisms. Remember if you are unsure of the quality of your water, get it tested.

Reverse osmosis units will not operate efficiently at water pressures below 40 – 45 psi.

Pre-filters and post-filters need to be re-placed on a regular basis. The length of time between changing pre-filters will depend on the water quality, especially the concentration of solids.

The good news for supporters of the reverse osmosis filtration system is that Gulf Oil and Eastman Kodak are spending resources to improve the present weakness of the reverse osmosis filtration system, particularly the membrane, to produce ultra clear high purity water low in dissolved solids, practically free from hardness components and essentially sterile.

Distilled Water
Distillation is the process whereby water is boiled, evaporated and the vapor condensed; leaving all chemicals, toxins and waste behind.

Distillation will remove bacteria, viruses, cysts, heavy metals, organics, in organics, and particulates.

Dr. Zoltan Rona and Dr. Gabriel Cousens, specializing

in natural health, have this to say about distilled water: "Drinking distilled water is useful for people seeking to cleanse or detoxify the body for short periods of time or working to heal a serious health challenge."

Other than this, Dr. Zoltan and Dr Gabriel do not recommend drinking distilled water for the following reasons:

- The more distilled water a person drinks, the higher the body acidity becomes. Natural health writers generally agree that the body maintains best health when it maintains a pH leaning to the alkaline side rather than the acidic side.

- The longer one drinks distilled water, the more likely the development of mineral deficiencies and an acid state.

- They advise against using distilled water when you are fasting because of the rapid loss of electrolytes (sodium, potassium, chloride) and trace minerals such as magnesium. The resulting deficiencies can cause heart beat irregularities and high blood pressure.

- Almost without exception, people who consume distilled water exclusively, eventually develop multiple mineral deficiencies.

On the other hand, well known personalities in natural health like Dr. Andrew Weil, Harvey & Marilyn Diamond, Paul Bragg, Norman Walker, Herbert Shelton and Dr. F. Batmanghelidj disagree:

- It is not true that distilled water leaches out minerals that have become part of your body's cell structure.

- Distilled water does not cause your teeth to deteriorate.

- As far as acidity goes, distilled water is close to a neutral pH and has no effect on the body's acid/base balance.
- The human body is designed to get its minerals from foods and not from drinking water.

Filtered Water
Your tap water is passed through a filter. The filter usually picks up suspended solids and minerals. After sometime in use, it becomes ineffective in removing suspended solids, and at the same time becomes a breeding ground for bacteria. This filtration system is unacceptable if you want purified water.

Mineral Water
It is your common bottled mineral water. Natural mineral water is pure and non-processed water from a subterranean source where it is bottled directly. There are over 3000 brands of mineral water commercially available worldwide.

Strictly speaking, water is water. The difference between various types of bottled waters lies mainly in where the source is located and the process the water goes through before it is sold to consumers. Not all bottled waters are recommended for drinking, so it is important to know the difference.

The U.S. FDA classifies mineral water as water containing at least 250 parts per million of total dissolved solids. No minerals may be added to this water.

Mineral water from natural springs commonly has a high content of calcium carbonate, magnesium sulfate, potassium, and sodium sulfate. It may also be impregnated with such gases as carbon dioxide or hydrogen sulfide.

The practice of taking mineral water for health still remains hugely popular in many countries. In the US, however, the FDA disallows advertisers to claim the health benefits of mineral water.

The choice to give your children bottled water or tap water is ultimately your own. The major problem is with the safety claims made about bottled water. Safety standards are actually often more rigorous for tap water than they are for bottled water.

CHOICE

The answer is clean spring water and water that has been filtered by reversed osmosis. I do not recommend drinking either tap or distilled water unless one is faced with a health challenge that requires mineral free clean water.

GOLD NUGGETS

"Water is the driver of nature." – Leonardo da Vinci

"Water and air, the two essential fluids on which all life depends, have become global garbage cans." – Jacques Cousteau (1910-1997)

"Water is the blood in our veins." – Levi Eshkol, Israeli Prime Minister, 1962

"Water is life's mater and matrix, mother and medium. There is no life without water." – Albert Szent-Gyorgyi

Chapter 8

Get Regular Check Up

I t is so normal for us to visit the doctor only when we feel there's something wrong. But the symptoms of most degenerative diseases today are silent and by the time it shows up, it may be too late to treat. So remember, it is not true that no symptoms mean your child is disease free. Healthy children are more likely to become healthy adults.

MEDICAL CHECK UP

If you want to bring up heart healthy happy and active children, parents are advised to subject their children to a five yearly general routine medical checkup. Their check up should generally include:

- A complete physical exam: A head-to-toe exam.

- Check their of growth and development.

- Make sure your child has up-to-date immunizations (shots) such as vaccine for hepatitis B vaccine, rotavirus, diphtheria, measles, mumps, rubella and others.

- Check their eyesight, hearing, teeth, nose, throat and abdominal area.

- Check their blood lipid profile to include their cholesterol, blood sugar and iron deficiency and liver function.

- Blood pressure numbers.

- Urine sample to check the health of their kidney.

Since a regular health checkup is indispensable, it is advisable to have a family doctor. A family doctor is the one you see for all your health issues. He holds all the medical records of your children for future reference.

Chapter 9

Get Them Off the Couch

The problem of obesity in children has more than doubled in the past thirty years. Although there are many contributing factors, a major cause: Our children are becoming more sedentary.

A SEDENTARY ISSUE

According to the Kaiser Family Foundation, the average American child today spends more than five hours a day or nearly 40 percent of their waking hours watching TV, playing video games, or sitting in front of a computer.

The school system must also take some of the blame. Many schools around the country are cutting back on physical activity and placing more emphasis on academic performance. This move has deprived many children of their major source of exercise as they spend a greater part of their lives in school.

The Lancet in its Oct. 26, 2001 issue reported that severely obese children suffer from stiff arteries, making them vulnerable to atherosclerosis in adulthood. Further, adult diseases such as high blood pressure and type 2 diabetes are affecting younger and younger children.

Obese children tend to be more sedentary than normal weight children.

The good news is that many studies have shown that physically active children are less likely to be obese as they grow into adulthood. Exercise is one of the most important key to better health.

The focus should be on getting exercise and at the same time having fun. If a child is sedentary or overweight, they may need to become physically active gradually.

As different children mature differently, find an activity that matches their maturity.

THE BENEFITS OF EXERCISE

Developing positive exercise habits is one of the most important gifts you can give to your children. Here are some good reasons why your child should exercise everyday:

• Exercise increases blood flow to the brain that makes a child more alert, helps to overcome stress, anxiety and depression.

• Exercise can help your child to sleep better and equip them to handle the physical and emotional challenges of life.

• Exercise can help your child age well. This may not seem important now but they will reap the reward as they grow to adulthood.

• Exercise helps build strong muscles and bones.

- Exercise helps build a leaner body because exercise helps control body fat.

- Exercise improves blood circulation and strengthens the heart.

- Exercise helps the lymph system to function at an optimal level as the lymphatic system relies on body movement, muscular stimulation and impact exercises such as jumping to remove toxins, germs, viruses, and bacteria from the body.

- Strengthens the immune system. The immune system is the body's defense mechanism against foreign invaders such as viruses, bacteria, fungi and even cancer cells.

- Physically active children have better bowel movement thus reducing the risk of constipation.

HOW MUCH EXERCISE IS ENOUGH?

Here are the current activity recommendations for kids, according to the National Association for Sport and Physical Education (NASPE):

Age	Minimum Daily Activity	Comments
Infant	No specific requirements	Physical activity should encourage motor development
Toddler	1½ hours	30 minutes planned physical activity and 60 minutes

		unstructured physical activity (free play)
Preschooler	2 hours	60 minutes planned physical activity and 60 minutes unstructured physical activity (free play)
School age	1 hour or more	Break up into bouts of 15 minutes or more

Here are some more views on how much exercise is enough for your children:

- Children under two should not watch television. For children over two years and older, watching television, playing video games or the computer should be limited to no more than one to two hours of quality program per day (Academy of Pediatrics).

- Children to exercise at least an hour a day, doing moderately intense activities, such as walking, swimming, or bicycling (The Institute of Medicine).

- All children 2 years and older should get at least 60 minutes of moderate to vigorous exercise on preferably all days of the week (Department of Health and Human Services (HHS).

- Children and young people who are currently inactive are advised to start with 30 minutes of exercise per day and gradually build this up to an hour.

Cardiovascular risk factors can be reduced and physical fitness enhanced with low to moderate levels of physical activity (40-60 percent of a person's maximal aerobic capacity) (Blair & Connelly, 1996).

• Current recommendations state that children and adults should strive for at least 30 minutes daily of moderate intensity physical activity (Pate, Pratt et al., 1995).

Most researchers feel that moderation is the key. Exercising at a moderate intensity should not make one gasping for breath. Ensure that your teen exercises vigorously at least 3 days per week.

HOW TO GET YOUR CHILDREN TO EXERCISE MORE?

• Be a good role model. The best way you can promote healthy exercise for your kids is to get involved in their activities.

• Talk to your children about the importance of physical activity.

• Get the kids involved in the family household or gardening chores.

• Consider enrolling your children in a club or exercise class such as martial arts, dancing or swimming.

• Parents must be strong enough to limit their children's sedentary activities such as sitting around the computer, TV or the internet.

GOLD NUGGETS

"Those who think they have no time for bodily exercise will sooner or later have to find time for illness." – Edward Stanley

"Lack of activity destroys the good condition of every human being, while movement and methodical physical exercise save it and preserve it." – Plato

"Fitness - if it came in a bottle, everybody would have a great body." – Cher

"The only exercise some people get is jumping to conclusions, running down their friends, side-stepping responsibility, and pushing their luck!" – Author Unknown

"Whenever I feel like doing exercise, I lie down until the feeling passes." – Robert M. Hutchins

"You will never find time for anything. If you want time, you must make it." – Charles Buxton

"Unless these are used, they will deteriorate. The human body is made up of some four hundred muscles; evolved through centuries of physical activity." – Eugene Lyman Fisk

We do not stop exercising because we grow old; we grow old because we stop exercising." – Dr. Kenneth Cooper, Cooper Institute

Chapter 10

Supplement
Your Children's Diet

Recent statistics show that a great majority of American children are not even eating up to the minimum Daily Value (DV) of nutrients, given our affluence and resources. It has been well said that many Americans dig their graves with their fork.

Many children today consume three out of five calories from fat or refined sugar. The result: Expanding waistlines, clogged arteries, and essential vitamins, minerals, and fiber are crowded out. No wonder, we have more obese and undernourished children than any time in the history of the world. The number of overweight and obese children in the United States has more than doubled since the 1960s.

The diseases we see later in the lives of your children such as heart attacks, strokes, high blood pressure, and cancer don't happen overnight. They are the result of a lifetime of poor lifestyle choices.

I want your children to have the best of health as they grow into adulthood, disease free. Good health is not just the absence of a major illness. It is the enjoyment of good food, with good digestion, proper utilization and elimination, clear skin, fine muscle tone, and maximum resistance to stress, infection, and fatigue. It is living life to the fullest. It is aging without getting old.

We often talk too much about the cost of good nutrition and too little about the cost of bad nutrition. I think this is obvious and profound. I still remember the saying that goes like this, "Don't use all your health to get your wealth and then use all the wealth to get back your health." Sounds familiar!

WHY SUPPLEMENT CHILDREN'S DIET?

Food Is Not As Nutritious As It Used to Be

Our freely chosen diets don't supply the amounts of nutrients that we need. Compared to the foods your ancestors ate a century ago, your food supply is highly processed and heavily laden with chemicals. Most of the manufactured foods you eat today are grown on nutrient depleted soils and food processing, shipping, and long shelf life, all take their nutritional toll.

And the change has definitely not been for the better. Your food, that were intended by nature to nourish your body for energy and building a stronger defense system against disease, has been depleted or stripped of its nutrients. Some manufacturers may compensate for this loss by "enriching" their products with vitamins and minerals. You need to replace the nutrients missing from our foods in one way or another.

Foods today are not generally designed with your health in mind. New foods such as beverages, breakfast cereals, condiments (salad dressing and barbecue sources), candy, gum and snacks of every kind you can imagine, are introduced yearly into the market place. These new products are made to look healthy and to cater for your taste bud.

Just remember this rule of thumb: The more processing a food goes through, the more nutrient value it loses. Any prolonged low level of nutrients undermines health and makes the body more vulnerable to infectious diseases and degenerative disorders.

Chemical Additives Incorporated Into Our Food

Chemicals are being added to our foods in increasing numbers. There are more than 3,000 direct and indirect chemical additives in our food today. Food manufacturers add chemical coloring additives for their product to look attractive. To increase shelf life they add preservatives and to make food tasty they add artificial sweeteners, salt and fats. How deceptive can you be?

By the use of these various additives, they can develop new foods to enhance consumer acceptability and feed our illusions about what looks and taste healthy. The great majority of these food additives have absolutely nothing to do with nutritional value but for monetary gain.

We don't yet know the long term effects of these chemicals on your bodies, but we do know that certain nutrients above the Daily Value (DV) can help protect you against some of the damages that they may cause.

Children's Food Choices Are Swayed by Multimedia Advertising

Multimedia advertising on food products is possibly the most dangerous assault to your children's health. Their goal is not to build your optimal health or nutrition. It is to coerce you into buying what tastes good, is convenient, is easy to prepare, and at the same time, might even seem healthy, or at least harmless. Sometimes, I think if they work hard enough, they could make us believe that the space walk on the moon is a fake and pro-wrestling is real!

They have successfully swayed your children to opt for refined foods, low in fiber, vitamins, minerals, enzymes, antioxidants but laden with the wrong fats, chemicals, sugar and salt. Today, your children grow up on colas and other fizzy drinks, greasy chips, cookies, French fries, hot dogs, bologna, hamburgers, doughnuts, chicken pie, and the list of greasy and fatty foods are endless. Once the children are hooked by the media, the parents are easy meat. Study after study shows that parents let their children make restaurant choices. All these foods will weaken their immune system.

Widespread Pollution

Pollutants are being released into our air and water, on a level unheard of in the past. Today, we talk casually about acid rain, fish kills, and toxic waste. What is this pollution doing to your health? Optimal nutrition may help protect you against some of the effects of widespread pollution.

Nutrients as Protector of Diseases

Your children need certain nutrients in higher levels than can be comfortably obtained in their day-to-day diets in order to prevent diseases. Some of the diseases, we used to blame on age itself are now being related to a lifetime of poor nutrition.

A growing volume of evidence indicates that proper consumption of certain vitamins and minerals can help prevent or delay the onset of chronic diseases, we mistakenly blame on age itself. Research shows that 90 percent of heart disease, 70 percent of cancer, 80 percent of cataracts, and 90 percent of high blood pressure are preventable by optimal nutrition and lifestyle modification.

Changing Food Choices and Habits

Our food choices and habits have changed dramatically in the past decades, unfortunately for the worse. We are now a nation of speed eaters and grazers. To find out let's take a test. This is a five question test to give you some idea just how well you and your family eat on a day-to-day basis.

1.   Do you sit down with your whole family present and have three home cooked meals a day?
2.   How about two home-cooked meals a day?
3.   One home-cooked meal a day with the family present?
4.   Think back yesterday, where did you eat and just how nutritious were the meals?

I have presented these questions to thousands of people, and the results are consistent. Americans, even informed Americans, just do not choose to consistently eat an optimal diet.

FOOD SUPPLEMENT IS NO LONGER AN OPTION

Heed the advice of Dr. Michael Janson, President of American Preventive Medicine Association. "If you live in a perfect world, in a perfect environment, eating a perfect diet and had perfect genes, you might still benefit from supplements."

If your children cannot or will not change their unhealthy diet, the answer is to add food supplements to their diet unless they live on a farm, far from urban pollution, where they can grow their own fruits and vegetables organically, raise all their own meat products, and have access to plenty of clean, spring water.

The point I want to make now is simply this: Supplements can help make up for shortcomings in the diet. There is no doubt in my mind that an inadequate diet plus a safe supplement program is certainly better than an inadequate diet alone. Of course, the best approach is a good diet, further energized by optimal supplementation. For many children, food supplements are no longer an option but a necessity, in today's toxic world. However, food supplements are not a substitute or excuse for poor dietary choices.

HOW TO BEGIN A FOOD SUPPLEMENT PROGRAM

What kind of supplement should we take? Food supplement has become a big business. The market place is crowded with hundreds of products vying for your dollars. How can you know which are the best products? How can you intelligently begin a food supplement program?

The Five Basics is the absolute minimum to begin a nutritional starter program for your children. This program fits the needs of nearly everyone and will not cost an arm or a leg. I strongly urge you and your family to give the Five Basics a trial. I cannot guarantee you will leap tall buildings in a single bound, but I can guarantee you will experience a noticeable difference in the way you feel.

Following which I will introduce the program I call the Plus Five. They are the rising stars that can possibly help to prevent the main killer diseases such as cancer and heart disease. Taking extra amounts of nutrients to help prevent chronic diseases is the frontier of nutritional science.

Together you have the "Basic Five plus Five." This will constitute an effective, health promoting, and important change in your nutritional well-being. What you choose from this category, will depend upon your children's individual needs and wishes.

Once again, please do try to eat a balanced diet, high in nutrient density but for insurance add the Basic Five plus Five supplements to fill in the gaps in your diet.

THE FIVE BASICS

The Multi-Vitamin Mineral (Multi)

This is the first nutrient to consider, since you are going to attempt to replace nutrients that may be short or missing in your children's diet; this is the logical place to begin. We need to establish our nutritional foundation on firm ground. Most health conscious physicians, dietitians, and nutritionists totally agree with this.

There are a lot of companies on the market today that are just after your money. They have little or no science behind their product, but they do have a lot of "hype" on the label and in their accompanying literature. It is difficult at times to separate the truth from the sales pitch.

Since the label is the first place to begin on your choice of company, I want to spend a little extra time to be sure you understand how to read these often complex labels.

I have looked at hundreds of labels of various multivitamins from a myriad of companies. As a result of this study, I developed some cautions to follow. This is not fool-proof, but you will at least be eliminating a lot of questionable products that are so prevalent on the market today.

- Check to be sure that all the nutrients with established US Daily Value (DV) are listed on the labels. A good multi should contain all 12 vitamins and 7 minerals clearly printed on the label. Count the nutrients listed on the multi label and make sure all 19 is there.

- Beware of lengthy, impressive labels. Some labels are quiet lengthy and impressive but they are often lacking in the U.S. DV, or they add fluff or cheap label lengtheners to the label. Usually these fluffs are non-essential nutrients marked with an asterisk. Omit them, as you count up the essential nutrients.

- Check the percents of the US DV present on the label. Each of the vitamins should be present in at least 100 percent of the DV. Any less and you are not looking at an adequate product. The mineral should also be 100 percent with the exception of calcium, magnesium and phosphorus.

- Watch out for sales hype on the label. For example some companies are claiming that their multi is formulated with cruciferous vegetables. These vegetable compounds look good on the label but they are present in small amounts to be of any benefit.

- A good multi should also have nine micronutrients such as selenium, manganese, chromium, molybdenum, nickel, tin, vanadium, boron and silicon.

- Read the company's literature. Many are just sales talk and not science. A good product will include clinical studies done on the product they are selling.

Protein

You are made of protein. Your hair, skin, muscle, ligaments, and tendons are protein. Many hormones and thousands of enzymes are protein. Your immune system is nearly all protein. Refer to chapter 4 for more information on proteins.

Probably most Americans think they get plenty of protein. After all, as a nation, we devour hundreds of thousands of pounds of beef, poultry, pork, and eggs each day.

Why then should we need a protein supplement?

The reason is that the protein sources Americans seem to favor also tend to be packed with large doses of fat and cholesterol which are risk factors for heart disease. Currently we get about 40 percent of your calories from fat. Most nutritionist advice us to limit our fat intake to 30 percent of total calories. For many people, this means cutting back on their favorite foods like hamburgers, pork chops, and steaks.

As you cut down on fats and cholesterol, you also cut down on protein. To compensate for the loss of protein in my low fat diet, I add a powdered soy protein supplement as insurance for my daily diet. The advantage of a complete, high quality soy protein supplement or meal replacement drink is that it can supply protein with no cholesterol and a minimum fat.

Supplementing your children's diet with soy protein has two added advantage. Firstly, soy contains saponins which have been reported to reduce serum cholesterol significantly. Secondly, it contains the nine essential amino acids in balanced amounts. All nine amino acids have to come together at one time, in sufficient amounts, for your body to utilize the protein effectively.

Adding a good quality soy protein drink to your children's usual diet is a simple, healthy, and convenient way to assure optimal intake of protein. Adequate complete, high quality protein is essential for life and health. Protein is just too important a nutrient for overall health to risk being even a little low.

Vitamin C
Most animals produce their own vitamin C but humans have to get this nutrient from the food we eat.

Vitamin C is extremely important to your children because it is involved in so many areas of health. The life-enhancing properties of vitamin C are too numerous to share here but I will highlight the important ones.

Vitamin C is needed for building and repairing bones, teeth, gums, and connective tissues. It is essential for the formation of collagen, a substance that gives structure to organs and muscles, tissues, bones, and cartilage.

Large doses of vitamin C can reduce the time you have a cold and can also reduce the unpleasant symptoms of a cold.

Vitamin C is a powerful water-soluble antioxidant and plays a vital role in protecting against free radical damage in the watery part of the cell of the body against degenerative diseases such as heart disease and cancer.

Vitamin C is needed to boost the immune system. Vitamin C's immune-enhancing effect makes it essential in fighting infection as well as in shortening the duration of an illness.

Vitamin C helps restore stress hormones. The more stress you have, the more C you need.

It is really quite easy to diagnose a true case of vitamin C deficiency. The classic symptom is scurvy, a disease that causes your gums to swell, your teeth to fall out, your wounds not to heal, and ultimately and if not treated, your death.

A good vitamin C supplement should come from natural sources and does not contain any preservatives, artificial flavors or coloring.

Vitamin C has to be consumed daily because the body does not store vitamin C. Pediatricians recommend that children should consume at least 30-45 mg of vitamin C per day. This is the minimum requirement to keep scurvy at bay but to raise disease free kids some nutritionists recommend a daily intake of 200 mg per day. If your child can consume the recommended daily allowance of five servings of fresh fruit or vegetables per day, they would be in this recommended target range.

B Complex
Like good family members, the B vitamins work more effectively together than separately. All of the B vitamins are water soluble. Prolonged physical or psychological stress that speeds up your metabolic rate can rob your body of the Bs. It is vital that they are replaced daily. There are eight recognized members of the B complex. To get them all, you must eat from a variety of foods such as whole grains, dark green vegetables and animal products each and every day.

If your children's diet mainly consists of processed and junk foods; they may not be getting enough of the B vitamins. If you do not have the needed B complex member available, you are not going to get proper energy release and they may experience tiredness and lower energy. Other symptoms include irritability, nervousness, depression, poor appetite, insomnia, constipation, poor hair quality and various skin problems.

Here is what you should look for when choosing a good quality B complex:

1. The product should contain eight recognized members of the B family. They are: Thiamin, Riboflavin, Niacin, B6, Folic acid, B12, Biotin and Pantothenic acid.
2. Six should be present in about 450 percent of the DV. However, Biotin and Folic acid should be at 100 percent of the DV.
3. It should not contain artificial colors, flavors or preservatives and sweeteners.
4. Preferably in tablet form.

Vitamin E and Selenium

The primary advantage of Vitamin E is that it helps to protect cell membranes (oily part) from the harmful oxidation of fatty acids. Unless these oxidants or free radicals are stopped they are like a bull loose in a china shop. They can blast through cell walls, damaging the ability of the cell to function effectively. Inside the cell, they can alter the DNA which can set up the cell for cancer.

Vitamin E also helps protect the walls of red blood cells and prevent its premature destruction. It aids in developing healthy blood circulation and new cell formation. It helps speed the healing of burns and open scars. Vitamin E is also an immune booster.

The DV is only 15 International units. Amounts needed for various protective effects in the scientific literature range from 100 to 800 IU.

Choose the natural source of Vitamin E. A natural source will be labeled d-alpha tocopherol. The synthetic version is labeled as dl alpha tocoperhol or l-alpha tocopherol.

A good natural vitamin E contains not only tocopherols such as gamma, alpha, and d-alpha but another family of compounds called tocotrienols which occur in nature with vitamin E.

Another ingredient is Selenium. Selenium and vitamin E work synergistically, each making the other potent. Taken together, vitamin E and selenium are much more powerful than each taken separately.

THE PLUS FIVE

Many people begin a food supplement program using the above Five Basics. Others may decide to add a program I call the Plus

Five to protect your children from certain degenerative diseases.

A Fiber Supplement

Adults only obtain about 50 percent of their required dietary fiber. If children are not eating lots of vegetables, fruits, cereals, and grains, chances are they are not getting enough fiber. Fiber is just as important for adults as well as children.

Most health scientists accept intestinal disorders, including cancer, as diseases that start in youth, but show up as we age. For example; the average age of onset for colonic cancer is about 55. These are diseases of age that start in youth.

If intestinal disorders are not enough, all diseases are made worse by a shortage of dietary fiber. These include heart disease, high blood pressure, and stroke. It seems that fiber is important at any age.

The question to follow all this is "how much?" In my opinion, children should be encouraged to obtain their fiber from natural sources such as fruits, grains, and vegetables. But most children today don't eat enough fibers on a regular basis, so it is appropriate to add two to four grams of a powdered fiber supplement to their food daily that contain both soluble and insoluble fiber. This can be accomplished by adding some in their cereal, in drinks, on vegetables, salads or on any food.

Besides Chapter 2, if you want more detail information on fiber, read my book entitled *Detox with Fiber.*

Eicosapentaenoic Acid (EPA)

There are two essential fatty acids namely omega-3 and omega-6 fatty acid from fats that our body cannot make, but must come from food. Fatty acids are building blocks for fats.

The most abundant food source of omega-3 fatty acid or EPA are found in cold oily ocean fish such as mackerel, sardines, salmon, haddock, anchovies, albacore tuna, herring and dogfish. Omega-3 fatty acid is also found in flaxseed.

The omega-6 fatty acid is found mainly in safflower, sunflower and corn. For the body to remain healthy, the ratio of omega-3 fatty acid to omega-6 fatty acid is an important consideration. Most researchers recommend a ratio of 2:1 in favor of omega-3 fatty acid.

If your children eat fish rich in EPA thrice a week, you are probably getting some EPA and DHA. However, as most children find fishy food not to their taste and have a significant imbalance of fats (too much omega-6 fats), it is worthwhile to consider taking a supplement containing EPA and DHA. It comes conveniently in capsules in dark brown bottles that usually contain 180 mg of EPA and 80 gm of DHA. To be certain your children are getting enough omega-3 fatty acid, give them one to three capsules daily.

For more details, see Chapter 3 where we discussed about EPA in greater detail.

Beta-Carotene

Beta-carotene is a precursor of vitamin A. It is sort of like having a reserve tank of vitamin A. Beta-carotene is superior to vitamin A in two ways:

Firstly, your body naturally can convert beta-carotene to vitamin A when the body needs and you will never run the risk of being short.

Secondly, vitamin A can be toxic when taken in excess but beta-carotene is a non toxic storage form of vitamin A even in large doses. When the body needs vitamin A, it converts beta-carotene into this valuable vitamin. Unlike vitamin A, beta-carotene is safe to take in higher doses.

Thirdly, like vitamins C and E, beta-carotene is also a powerful antioxidant that works in the oily part of the cell membrane. In dozens of studies, high levels of beta-carotene have being shown to be protective against the development of cancers in at least ten sites in the body.

Beta-carotene's power does not stop here. It can also help prevent cataracts, slow the wrinkling or early aging of the skin, prevent night blindness, help cells produce mucous and enhances the immune system by improving the function of the white blood cells.

If your children eat a medium serving of orange or red vegetables every day; two green leafy vegetables every day; and some fruit with colored flesh daily every day, your kid is in good shape. The problem is that very few children consistently eat this way.

The benefits of beta-carotene to your children's health and well-being are just too great to run the risk of low levels of this powerful nutrient. I recommend your children to take at least 10,000 I.U. of beta-carotene daily.

Garlic

This is the most widely accepted and used of all herbs. Garlic has a two thousand year history of proven success on a consistent basis. From Hippocrates to the era of modern medicine, garlic has been used as "nature's antibiotic."

It fights off bacterial infections especially those of the throat, ears, mouth, sinuses, and bronchial tubes. Garlic can slow or kill more than 60 fungi and 20 types of bacteria. It seems to work by enhancing the immune system.

Another big plus for garlic is that bacterial resistance does not develop as it does when antibiotics are used. It worked so well that a license was issued for garlic by the Ministry of Health in the United Kingdom.

It also allows manufacturers of garlic products to claim that it is traditionally used for the treatment of all the inflammatory and respiratory problems I just mentioned.

Garlic works to improve the number of risk factors in heart disease. It consistently lowers cholesterol by 10 to 20 percent and decreases triglycerides. In addition, it lowers blood pressure, reduces edema and causes the blood to flow more smoothly. By the way, in Germany, garlic is a licensed medicine for coronary artery disease.

Calcium

Calcium helps your nerves conduct impulses, allows your muscle to contract, aids your blood to coagulate properly so wounds can heal quickly and assists in maintaining normal blood pressure.

Calcium also produces and activates numerous hormones and enzymes, stabilizes and maintains cell membranes, regulates heartbeat, aids in sleep and stress and helps prevent gum diseases and stress fractures.

Calcium is the most common mineral in the body. Around 99 per cent of the calcium in the body is found in the bones or skeleton; the rest is in teeth, soft tissues and blood. The skeleton is a living tissue and acts as a calcium reservoir, which needs to be topped up daily. A high intake of dietary calcium is essential for growth of strong bones and teeth.

Calcium, phosphorus and vitamin D work together in the body to achieve the right calcium levels that your body needs. Your body uses vitamin D to help transport calcium to your bones.

Severe calcium deficiency can result in diseases like rickets in children and osteoporosis later in life. Osteoporosis can lead to fragile bones and an increased risk of fractures.

Here is a recommended intake by The National Institutes of Health Expert Panel, 1994 Consensus Conference:

Children 1-5 years .... 800 mg
      6-10 years .... 800 – 1,200 mg
Adolescent / Young Adults
      11- 24 years .... 1,200 – 1,500 gm

Unfortunately, many national nutrition surveys show that most teen girls and almost half of teen boys are not getting the recommended amount of calcium they need.

My suggestion is to use a calcium magnesium supplement that also contain phosphorus and vitamin D. Calcium should be taken with a meal. It absorbs better that way. Calcium carbonate or ground limestone is an excellent source of calcium. It has been used as a supplement for decades with excellent results.

WINNING THEM OVER

Explain carefully the reasons and the benefits of supplementation. Educate your child on how nutrients will help them to grow up strong, healthy, and beautiful. Show your child how and when to take supplements. Ask for suggestion. Get your child involved.

Accept your child's feeling. Back off if necessary and introduce the supplement at another time. Give children choices.

Appreciation and praise can reinforce co-operation and enthusiasm. Hug and kisses always work!

Teach through role modeling. Children will imitate what you do or don't do. Therefore, if you are not supplementing your diet or making changes in your lifestyle, don't expect children to be willing to obey just because you say so.

Recognize and realize that you are the authority and the

key person responsible for the success of your family's health. If you are not going to take any positive steps to encourage your children to supplement their food, no one else will.

CLOSING COMMENTS

Given the world we live in today, I suggest you begin with the Five Basics. The Five Basic nutrients can form the basis of your children personal health program. Together with the Plus Five, they will constitute an effective, health promoting, and important change in their nutritional well- being.

Once again, please try to get your children to eat a balanced diet, high in nutrient density, but for "health insurance," do add good quality food supplements to fill in the gaps.

GOLD NUGGETS

"When you take just enough of a nutrient to supply for your body's needs, you are taking at a nutritional dose. You can take them at a level that greatly exceeds your nutritional needs. This is described as a "therapeutic dosage." – Steven Bratman, M.D.

"As far as we know, early civilization did not use vitamin and mineral supplements. So why have supplements become necessary now? The reason lies in the dramatic changes in our lifestyle and technology, especially over the last decades. Essentially, we have polluted not only our air and water, but our food as well, while taking a great deal of nutrition out of it." – Dr. Duke Johnson, M.D.

Chapter 11

Coach Your Children to Manage Stress

Anything that poses a challenge or a threat to the well-being of your children is a stress. Stress affects their body as much as food and exercise. Stress can trigger their body's response to perceived threat or danger, the "fight-or-flight response." However, whether the stress can hurt their body, depends greatly on their response to it.

Stress causes their body to release two important hormones, cortisol and adrenaline to heightened muscle preparedness, increase their heart rate, sweating, and alertness to protect them from the impending challenge, they are facing. Non-essential body functions slow down, such as their digestive and immune systems when they are in fight-or-flight response mode. All resources can then be concentrated on rapid breathing, blood flow, alertness and muscle use.

WHAT IS STRESS?

Stress is a normal and necessary part of life. Different children react differently to stressful experiences. However, not all stress experiences are negative. When stress is experienced for an extended period (chronic stress) it can affect their school work and also their relationship with their peers and family. In this situation, parental assistance is absolutely necessary.

While you want to manage or eliminate the negative types of stress in your children, you also want to keep positive forms of stress intact. Without it, life would be extremely dull and depression would be rampant, so relief from *all* stress isn't the best goal.

Types of Stress
There are a few different types of stress that your children may encounter.

Eustress
It is basically a desirable form of stress which is healthy. This type of stress is fun and exciting. Some examples include skiing down a slope or excitement of winning a race, joy experienced on a roller-coaster ride or accomplishing a challenge.

Acute Stress
A very short-term type of stress that is either positive or more distressing. This is the type of stress your children most often encounter in their day-to-day life. Meeting datelines, over exertion, minor accidents are some examples of acute stress.

Chronic Stress
This type of stress seems never-ending and inescapable. Taking too many responsibilities, over-worked, and always in a hurry, are some examples. This type of stress is perhaps the greatest enemy to your children's energy, vitality and well-being.

What Causes Stress in Children?
There are many causes of stress and here are some: Family conflict, pressure of school work, tests and examinations,

moving house, abuse, fear of failure, starting school or childcare, birth of a new baby, illness, separation or divorced parents, job change, moving to a new location, loss of a pet, death of a family member.

Stress affects the body in many different ways. Some of these are obvious, but others may not be as noticeable or easy to detect until they become more severe. Different people are affected more or less intensely, and in different ways. There is no one right way to cope with stress. Managing and reducing stress requires hard work from both parents and children. Here are some common signs that indicate that your child is under stress:

Physical Stress: If they show signs such as diarrhea, sweaty hands, perspiration, rapid breathing or having nightmare, headache, backache, muscle tension and stiffness, nausea, dizziness, insomnia, rapid heartbeat, chest pain, weight gain or loss, skin breakouts such as hives and eczema and frequent colds.

Emotional Stress: If they show signs such as lack of interest, irritability, depression, anger, crying, jealousy, overly critical of others, nightmares, insomnia, or changes in eating habits (either increased or decreased), often confused about situations, or more hostile than usual, moodiness, restlessness, short temper, impatience, feeling tense and on "edge," feeling overwhelmed, sense of loneliness and isolation and general unhappiness.

Behavioral Stress: If they show signs of wanting to be alone, nervous habits such as nail biting or pacing, suffer increase or decrease in appetite and lacking energy or being clingy, sleeping too much or too little, procrastination, neglecting responsibilities, teeth grinding or jaw clenching, overdoing activities, overreacting to unexpected problems and picking fights with others.

Cognitive Stress: Memory problems, indecisiveness, inability to concentrate, trouble thinking clearly, poor judgment, seeing only the negative, anxious or racing thoughts, constant worrying, loss of objectivity and fearful anticipation.

MANAGING STRESS

Here are some effective ways you can use to help your children grow up to manage stress:

Sharpen Their Relational Skills

As parents, it is important to nurture your children to develop relational/emotional skills with people. These characteristic traits are a strong antidote for stress as most of the problems in life arise out of dealing with people. Poor relational skills will lead to chronic stress. There are several ways you can help your children build their relational skills:

1. Love people

Instill in children loving thoughts about people. What they need to do is to look beyond people's faults and see their needs. Then they can begin to love people. Every human being has some goodness in them. Expect the best in people. Into their personality built the following qualities:

Forgiveness: This is the ability to release someone who has wronged them. Teach them to let go off the past and to get on with the present by forgiving people who hurt them. The people in the past cannot hurt them unless they allow them to do so. Life is too short to hold a grudge.

Courtesy: Treat others as they would like to be treated.

Courtesy is good manners and polite behavior. The best way to be courteous is to think of every person they encounter as their friend. Ingrain in the mind of your children this old but wise saying: "Don't do onto others what you don't want others to do onto you," and they will not go wrong when it comes to dealing with people.

Humility: Put others people's interests before their own. Humility is not thinking less of oneself, but thinking of oneself less.

Generosity: Is the giving of their time, abilities, and money to help others.

Honesty: Be true to themselves and others.

2. Be Joyful

Joy is more than happiness. Joy is an attitude. Joy makes live enjoyable and it is a strong antidote to stress.

All problems have a purpose and value, as problems help your children to develop perseverance, character and hope. Problems in their life help them to mature. This can only take place when they choose to be joyful in times of stress. When they have this kind of mindset, they will realize that there are positive things behind all the bad things that happen.

To be joyful, guide them to develop an attitude of gratitude. Hans Seyle, the father of stress says that gratitude produces more emotional energy than any other attitude in one's life. People who are grateful are the happiest people around. Your children should be surrounded by friends who have a positive attitude in life.

Cultivate inner joy by "giving" instead of "taking" all the time. Focus and concentrate on helping others. Volunteer their services without being asked. When they start loving others they will also feel joy in their lives.

3. Develop Relational Peace With God and With Others

When there is peace, one can be calm and content on the inside and don't have anger towards others. Your children need relational peace. Relational conflict can be a strong cause of stress. Many children experience relationship problems with their teacher, their family, friends and relatives. Relational peace reduces conflict. Conflicts, competition and criticism lead them to worry and rob their peace. They should learn to forgive people. Guilt is the number one destroyer of peace.

4. Develop Patience

Patience means one is willing to wait for a while to get what one wants without becoming anxious or angry. The real test of patience comes not in waiting for something to happen, but in how one acts while waiting.

Impatience is a lack of peace. When your children have peace in their heart, almost nothing can make them become impatient. Their patience level drops to zero when they become angry. They must be able to put up with things that they do not agree with; without losing their cool. Patience begins by changing the way they look at people or circumstances. They must acknowledge that they are not perfect then it will be easier to accept the imperfections of others.

Here are some quotations you can use to teach your children about patience:

"Patience is the companion of wisdom." – Saint Augustine.

"Patience is the ability to count down before you blast off." – Author Unknown.

"Patient is the best remedy for every trouble." – Titus Maccius.

"One moment of patience may ward off great disaster. One moment of impatience may ruin a whole life." –Chinese Proverb.

"If you are patient in one moment of anger, you will escape a hundred days of sorrow." – Chinese Proverb.

"Patience is the key to paradise." – Turkish Proverb.

5. Develop Kindness Into Their Character
Kindness is having sympathy and understanding for others and showing concern for those in need. This may be done though actions or just simple words of encouragement. Don't talk about people behind their backs and learn to smile at everyone, even if they are strangers.

A kind person has the following characteristics: Sensitive to others, supportive, sympathetic, candid and spontaneous to help when a situation arises.

6. Develop Gentleness into Their Character
Gentleness is being kind, friendly and tender to people instead of been harsh, rash, angry, or rough whom they come in contact with. They can do this by being understanding and not demanding.

Be gracious, not judgmental. Handle people who disagree with gentleness. Be teachable. Learn to admit when they are wrong. Handle a hurt without retaliating. When they are gentle to people they meet, they will feel good about themselves. They will develop a healthy esteem. A gentle response tends to create fewer enemies, and more friends.

7. Teach Self Control

A lot of children's stressful situations are caused by lack of self-control. The word refers to the *control of one's emotions, speech, desires, or actions by one's own will.* For instance, one lacks self control when one retaliates to an insult or unfair statement. One loses their cool.

The truth is self-control is a choice. Tell your children that the only way they can develop self control is to believe that they can change. Self control leads to confidence and inner sense of security. Here are some other ways you can help your children to learn self control:

Tell your children that although they cannot control what happens to them, but they can control their attitude towards what happens to them.

Even if you don't agree with their reasoning for losing their self control, some simple comments like, "That must be really hard for you," will go a long way toward opening that communication with your child.

Listen quietly without becoming defensive. Ask your child to tell you what's wrong. Listen attentively and calmly – with interest, patience, openness, and caring. Avoid any urge to judge, blame, lecture, or say what you think your child should have done instead.

Be a model of self-control. As parents if you often lose self-control and start yelling and swearing around the house, you're not setting a good example for your child. The best way to teach self-control is to demonstrate it at all times.

Be consistent in your rules or enforcements. As hard as it may be at times, be consistent and enforce the rules each time your child breaks one of them. When you're inconsistent, you're giving your child mixed signals. This means that your child is unclear as to what's expected of them and they may lose their self control.

8. Faithfulness

Faithfulness is a rare quality. It means to be reliable, trustworthy and dependable.

If these eight qualities are edged into the lives of your children, they will be able to cope with stress better as poor human relational skills can be a major cause of misery and chronic stress.

Expecting Too Much From Your Children

Parents often have great expectations of their children to excel in their studies and sports. Enrolling their children in too many activities may also cause unnecessary stress and frustration. You must allow your children to play and relax after school.

Time Management

Children must be taught time management. Teach them how to use a daily planner. This will help them to prioritize their activity to enable them to decide what activity they should get involved in and which ones to drop. In so doing, they are in control of their time. This ensures that they can have more time to relax outside of their studies.

Personal Freedom

You need to give your children every opportunity to make their decisions on their own, develop their negotiating skills, plan their own activities and experience the fruits of success and failures. Over controlled children will be ill prepared to cope with the outside world when they leave home.

Take Children's Fears Seriously

Do not force a child to be brave. Respect their feelings and try to understand them. Do not show anger or ridicule. Avoid saying something like: "It's silly to be scared." Telling children that it's alright to be scared is comforting to them. Reassure them they are safe.

Exercise: The Ultimate Stress Reliever

Make exercise and recreation a family affair. There is a lot of truth to the old saying, "Families that play together, stay together." If your children see you exercise, they are more likely to take it up themselves and continue this good habit into their adulthood years. Children who exercise regularly are more able to handle the long-term effects of stress or burnout. According to experts, children should do at least 90 minutes of exercise each day.

Regular exercise not only strengthens physical health but also benefits the mind and body. Exercise can cause release of chemicals called endorphins into their blood stream. This gives them an overall sense of well-being.

Kids who participate in sports or other forms of exercise have the opportunity to develop strong, healthy bodies, making them less inclined to worry excessively about how they measure up to others.

In addition to offering relief from unpleasant emotions, regular exercise can help kids and teens to improve their self-image and boost confidence.

Good Night's Sleep

Sleep deprivation is one of the leading causes of stress. And stress is one of the leading causes of insomnia. It is important to maintain a regular sleep routine, avoiding large meals just before sleeping. It is also important to avoid exercise just before sleep time.

In a stress free environment children sleep better, perform better, waken naturally and have energy and enthusiasm to face life.

Good Nutrition

Good nutrition optimizes the way the mind and body works. Nutrition affects their emotions, their ability to concentrate and to prevent illness, to grow and to develop into a healthy adult.

Stress can also affect both their digestion and their intake of nutrients, robbing them of key nutrients their body needs to grow.

The key is to improve your children's diet by replacing processed foods with unrefined wholesome food. You need to nourish them with vegetables and fruits, whole grains, pulses, lean meat and low fat dairy product.

Watch out for foods that are heavily laden with fats, sugar, salt and chemicals such as preservatives, coloring and additives.

A healthy diet gives your child the energy to handle daily stress, and keeps their blood sugar levels stable so they don't experience mood swings due to low blood sugar levels. Skipping meals and making poor food choices can contribute to fatigue, greater susceptibility to illness, greater feelings of stress, and a general feeling of poor health.

You may be able to reduce their stress by changing their diet. Foods and beverages that are helpful can be found in many stores. Herbal teas such as chamomile and peppermint have a calming effect. Vitamin B6 is an antidote for stress. Citrus fruits, bell peppers and baked potatoes are rich in vitamin C, which help the human body to maintain resistance to infection when under stress.

GOLD NUGGETS

"Worry is the senseless process of cluttering up tomorrow's opportunities with left over problems from today." – Barbara Johnson.

"It's easy to put off unpleasant tasks until "later." A far better strategy is this: Do the unpleasant work first so you can enjoy the rest of the day." – Family Christian Story.

"Stress is not what happens to us. It is our response to what happens. And response is something we can choose." – Maureen Killoran.

"When you find yourself stressed, ask yourself one question. Will it matters in 5 years from now. If yes, then do something about the situation. If not, then just let it go." – Catherine Pulsifer.

"Brain cells create ideas. Stress kills brain cells. Stress is not a good idea." – Frederick Saunders.

"Forgiveness doesn't make the other person right, it makes you free." – Stormie Omartian.

"If you judge people, you have no time to love them." – Mother Teresa.

Chapter 12

Teach Your Child
about Lifestyle Diseases

S anitation and medical advancement have brought infectious disease under control. Today, we are plagued by a whole new set of diseases caused by lifestyle and diet, unrelated to germs.

Parents must find ways to teach their children about diet and lifestyle related diseases as early as possible. This sounds odd but research has shown that most diseases have their roots in childhood. Obesity that once affected adults is now found in younger children in alarming numbers. Hypertension, heart disease and diabetes are now also affecting younger children and the numbers are growing year by year. We need a new approach if you want to raise disease free kids.

Good health does not come easy; you have to earn it. Unfortunately, many parents are too busy to have time allocated to look after the health of their children until they are faced with a major crisis. It is much easier to prevent a disease before it happens than to try to regain back health once it is lost. Prevention is a better option.

Since there are many lifestyle diseases, I want to focus just on a few major ones that are responsible for most of the deaths and disabilities that young and old suffer in the United States today.

LIVE STYLE RELATED DISEASE

Let's begin with the major lifestyle diseases of the 21st century that can endanger your children's health.

Heart Disease

If there is only one thing you can do for your child's well being, it is to teach them to love their heart. Heart disease (heart attack and stroke) is the number one killer in America.

Three of the biggest threats to heart health that trace back to childhood are pre-hypertension, pre-diabetes and obesity.

Pre-hypertension

Pre-hypertension is a precursor of hypertension or in simple plain language, the early stage of high blood pressure. Pre-hypertension is a warning sign or a wake up call. Left untreated, pre-hypertension is likely to progress to hypertension. The word hypertension is the medical word for high blood pressure.

"The whole purpose of using the term pre-hypertension is to encourage people to do what they can to reduce their risk for cardiovascular disease and to avoid having to use blood pressure medications. Everyone needs to be aware of their blood pressure level, particularly those with a family history of high blood pressure," says Daniel Jones, M.D., a hypertension expert in Jackson, Miss., and a spokesperson for the American Heart Association (AHA).

Blood Pressure

Blood pressure is the force of blood against the walls of arteries, as blood flows through the body. When blood pressure stays elevated over time, it is called *high blood pressure.*

Blood pressure is expressed in millimeters of mercury

(mm Hg). As the heart pumps, the vessels most affected are the arteries. Pressure in the arteries is our "blood pressure." Blood pressure is made up of two numbers: Systolic and diastolic (both from Greek words meaning contract and relax, respectively).

Systolic blood pressure is the pressure in the arteries. The first, or upper, number measures the pressure in your arteries when your heart beats (systolic pressure). The second, or lower, number measures the pressure in your arteries between beats (diastolic pressure). If your systolic pressure is 120 and your diastolic is 80, it would be written as 120/80 or spoken as "one-twenty over eighty."

Pre-hypertension is a systolic pressure from 120 to 139 or a diastolic pressure from 80 to 89. The diastolic blood pressure is an important number for younger people. The higher the diastolic blood pressure the greater the risk for heart attacks, strokes and heart failure.

The National Heart, Lung, and Blood Institute (NHLBI) have set a new "pre-hypertension" level of any reading above 120 over 80 as part of its new guidelines for the prevention, detection, and treatment of high blood pressure. We also now know that damage to arteries begins at fairly low blood pressure levels; those formerly considered normal and optimal.

For more information on high blood pressure, read my book entitled *7 Keys to Bring Your Blood Pressure Under Control.*

Pre-Diabetes

Pre-diabetes is a condition of high insulin levels, high triglycerides, low HDL cholesterol, insulin resistance, a growing waistline and blood glucose levels that are higher than normal but not high enough to be diagnosed as diabetes. You are in the grey zone between "normal" and "diabetic".

This is the first stage of diabetes, just like pre-hypertension is the first stage of hypertension. Pre-diabetes is sometimes also described as "borderline diabetes."

This condition that precedes diabetes was formerly described by a number of names such as metabolic syndrome (Syndrome X, insulin resistance syndrome), impaired glucose tolerance or impaired fasting glucose. The American Diabetes Association has officially adopted the term pre-diabetes, "as a wake-up call."

Symptoms of pre-diabetes develop so gradually that most people affected often don't recognize it. The damage to your micro-vascular (small blood vessels) and macro-vascular (large blood vessels) and vital organs like your heart, kidneys and eyes are already taking place at this stage because of the high insulin level in the blood caused by your body cells being insensitive to your insulin.

Pre-diabetes is far easier to turn around in the early stages than diabetes but, unfortunately, most people don't know that they have this condition until diagnosed with type 2 diabetes.

How Do You Know If You Have Pre-diabetes?
This is done by taking a blood sample in the morning after fasting for at least 12 hours or more the night before. Plain water is allowed during the fast. This is called a fasting glucose test.

Your insulin is beginning to lose its control over your blood sugar level if your reading exceeds 5.5 mmol/L. This is a sign of insulin resistance. See Table 1.

Table 1

Reading (mmol/L)	Diagnosis
From 3.9 to 5.5	Normal
From 5.6 to 5.5	Pre-diabetes
From 7 and above	Diabetes

For more details on pre-diabetes, read my book entitled, *7 Keys to Arrest and Reverse Life-threatening Pre-Diabetes.*

OVERWEIGHT AND OBESITY

According to the Centers for Disease Control and Prevention (CDC) American society has become "obesogenic." We are living in an age of excessive food intake, non-healthful foods, and physical inactivity.

Besides psychological damage, obesity is a health hazard and not just merely a cosmetic issue.

According to CDC, children who are overweight during childhood have an increased risk of obesity in adulthood and are at greater risk of developing degenerative diseases such as diabetes, high blood pressure and heart disease.

Childhood obesity is a problem, but you can turn it around if you accept that your children's health is largely in your hands. The greater the interests you show in your child's health, the more influence you will have over your child.

Today children are spending less of their leisure time exercising and more time watching TV, playing computer, or video-game. The rat race has been a major obstacle for many working parents to prepare nutritious, home-cooked meals. Fast food seems to be the order of the day in many homes. Obesity and overweight are major health issues that all parents must address if they want their children to grow up, disease free.

A study by researchers at Washington University School of Medicine in St. Louis, has found that children who are obese or who are at risk for obesity show early signs of heart disease similar to obese adults with heart disease.

Helping your children lead healthy lifestyles begins with you. Physically active parents who encourage nutritionally balanced meals at the dinner table and exercise consistently can instill lifelong healthy habits in their children.

Obesity versus Weight Loss

The location of fat is a more reliable indicator of your children's health than just their weight you see on the weighing scale. Excess body fat is the true cause of obesity.

Being overweight and obese does not mean the same thing. A person can be overweight without being obese (e.g. bodybuilder) but an obese person is always overweight. Overweight and obesity have only one thing in common: That is excess body weight.

Overweight people have excess body fat from muscles, bones, fat or body water while obese people have excess body fat especially around the abdomen, waist, hips and thighs.

What Do People Say about Obesity?

"While approximately one in every 400 children and adolescents have Type I diabetes; recent Government reports indicate that one in every three children born in 2000 will suffer from obesity, which as noted is a predominant Type II precursor." – Tim Holden.

"This might be the first generation where kids are dying

at a younger age than their parents and it is related primarily to the obesity problem." – Judy Davis.

"The rate of childhood obesity is just ridiculous. Anytime I can get involved with teaching them how to get physical exercise, I want to help in any way possible." – Shannon Miller.

"Childhood obesity is best tackled at home through improved parental involvement, increased physical exercise, better diet and restraint from eating." – Bob Filner.

"I couldn't open up a magazine, you couldn't read a newspaper, and you couldn't turn on the TV without hearing about the obesity epidemic in America." – Morgan Spurlock.

"More than ever, we as parents and a nation must do something about the growth of obesity in our children. We must do more than just talk, we must be concerned enough to act." – Lee Haney.

MEASURING OBESITY

Many experts are now suggesting that it's time to forget about losing total weight and instead to focus on how to reduce the fat especially around the waist or abdomen.

A child with a healthy weight but with a large abdomen is at a higher risk of weight-related diseases than a child who is overweight but with a small waist or abdomen.

There are several measurements you can use to determine whether you are obese or overweight. Each method has its pros and cons.

Body Mass Index (BMI)
For adults, overweight and obesity ranges are determined by using a number called the "Body Mass Index" (BMI). This

index is used to determine whether your body weight is appropriate for your height. To calculate your BMI divide your weight by the square of your height. For example, if I'm about 5'7" weighing 140lbs. I would have a BMI of 22.

The National Institute of Diabetes and Digestive and Kidney Diseases (NIDDK), use the following guidelines to define BMI:

- A BMI of less than 18.5 is considered underweight.
- A BMI of 18.5 to 24.9 is considered healthy.
- A BMI *of* 25 to 29.*9* is considered overweight.
- A BMI of 30 or more is considered obese.
- A BMI of 40 or greater is considered extreme obesity

BMI is not a perfect measure of body fat. For example, a very muscular person may have a high BMI without being overweight. The extra muscle adds to a person's body weight. BMI is usually a good indicator but is not a direct measurement of body fat.

Because the BMI focuses on excess weight than on where fats are distributed in the body, experts recommend that measuring the waist circumference or the waist-to-hip ratio could be used as additional tools to identify children at increase risk of overweight or obese related illness.

Waist Measurement
Waist measurement addresses only the circumference of the waist (distance around the waist). Waist circumference is a measure of the fat around the abdomen and a better indicator of your child's health status, even when the BMI shows that their weight is within a healthy range.

According to the World Health Organization, a male child is considered to be obese if his waist circumference is more than 90 cm (35.4 inches) and for a female child if she exceeds 80 cm (31.5 inches)

Waist-to-Hip Ratio

Using a measuring tape to check your waist-to-hip ratio is another way of judging whether your weight is healthy. The waist-to-hip ratio refers to the comparison of weight carried between your waist and hips. Waist-to-hip ratio is a simple measure of where fat is distributed in your body. The waist-to-hip ratio is a measure of abdominal obesity.

To determine your waist-to-hip ratio, use a measuring tape to measure the narrowest part of the waist and the widest part of the hip. Divide the waist measurement by the hip measurement. This gives you your child's waist-to-hip ratio.

Waist-to-Hip Ratio Chart

Male	Female	Health Risk
less than 0.9	less than 0.80	Low Risk
0.9 to 0.99	0.8 to 0.89	Moderate Risk
1.0+	0.9+	High Risk

Waist-to-hip ratio is a better predictor of heart attack risk than calculating a person's body mass index, say researchers who studied people in 52 countries.

If waist-to-hip ratio is used to define obesity instead of the traditional BMI, the number of children at risk of heart attack is three times what doctors currently estimate, say researchers.

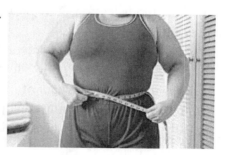

To reduce your waist-to-hip ratio, it is important to decrease abdominal fat and to maintain muscle mass through strengthening exercises. People who have more muscle mass tend to have larger hip circumferences, and thus a lower waist-to-hip ratio.

For further reading on obesity, read my book entitled: "Escape the Obesity Trap: Overcome Your Body's Resistance to Permanent Weight Loss."

CANCER

The National Cancer Institute estimates that at least 80 percent of all cancer in America has to do with lifestyles. The authoritative Journal *Nutrition Today* stated: "Since it is thought that up to 50 percent of all cancers may be influenced by diet, dietary modification may have a dramatic impact on this disease."

So as responsible parents do not hesitate take positive steps to alter your children's lifestyle while they are growing up and you will dramatically alter their chances of contracting cancer when they grow into adulthood. Many experts believe that 50 percent or more of all cancers in America is attributable to what we eat or do not eat.

The war against cancer is a winnable war. Early detection is great. We just need to change tactics from seeking the "magic bullet" cure to aggressively pursuing prevention. There are literally hundreds of valid studies proving the power of diet, modification, and proper food supplements on cancer prevention.

Consider this statement from Dr. John C. Bailor of the Harvard School of Public Health, "The main conclusion we draw is that some 35 years of intensive effort focused largely on improving treatment must be judged a qualified failure. The reasons for this failure need to be carefully assessed, but in the meanwhile, it may be our approach to cancer that needs to be changed. The most promising areas are in prevention."

EATING DISORDERS

An eating disorder is a medical condition that requires professional medical attention and treatment. For most children, eating disorders begins when they are 11 to 13 years old. They are more common among girls. Unfortunately, many kids and teens hide these disorders from their parents.

Forms of Eating Disorder

There are two major forms of eating disorder:

- **Bulimia:** This is characterized by habitual binge eating and purging. A child with bulimia may experience weight fluctuations, but rarely experiences the low weight associated with anorexia.

- **Anorexia nervosa:** To control their weight, the child goes on starvation and purge by vomiting or taking laxatives.

What Causes Eating Disorders?

It is not clear what causes eating disorder. It is possible that a combination of factors such as psychological, genetic, social and family factors may be the cause. For example sports such as ballet and gymnastics are possible contributors because of its emphasis on leanness. Some research suggests that media images of beautiful slim women from television and movies can contribute to the rise in the incidence of eating disorders.

Effects of Eating Disorder

A child with anorexia or bulimia may experience dehydration and other medical complications. If left untreated, it can affect the brain and cause symptoms such as dizziness, fainting, agitation, confusion, inability to concentrate, and loss of memory.

Anorexia may affect a child's growth, her bone mass, puberty delays, an irregular heartbeat, blood pressure, severe inflammation of the esophagus, in addition to gastric disturbances and erosion of tooth enamel.

Teens with bulimia often exhibit behavioral problems such as shoplifting, sexual promiscuity including drug and alcohol abuse.

HOW CAN YOU HELP

It's common for kids with eating disorders to act defensive and angry when confronted with their eating disorder.

Instead, approach your child about your concerns in a loving, supportive and non-threatening manner. Show your child that you love him or her for who she is and what she does, not how she looks.

Get your child to be involved in the preparation of healthy, nutritious meals on a consistent basis.

GOLD NUGGETS

"If you don't take care of yourself, the undertaker will overtake that responsibility for you." – Carrie Lat.

"A man too busy to take care of his health is like a mechanic too busy to take care of his tools." – Spanish proverb.

"Brain cells come and brain cells go, but fat cells live forever." – Author Unknown.

"The older you get, the tougher it is to lose weight, because by then your body and your fat are really good friends." – Author Unknown.

"Sickness is the vengeance of nature for the violation of her laws." – Charles Simmons.

"It is a hard matter, my fellow citizens, to argue with the belly, since it has no ears." – Plutarch.

Chapter 13

Minimize Exposure to
Toxic Chemicals at Home

Chemicals play a major role in the health of your children. Some chemicals have immediate toxic effects. Others are toxic to our bodies only after repeated, long-term exposure. Children are vulnerable to the exposure of these chemicals because of their immature immune system.

As this a very broad subject, I will briefly touch on the more harmful chemicals as childhood exposure to these toxic chemicals at home and in their food, over time, can affect their health in later part of their adult lives.

TOXIC CHEMICALS IN FOOD

Hormones and Antibiotics in Animal Protein

Today artificial hormones are used in animals to make them grow faster as well as to increase milk production. The hormone residues found in meat and milk products, poses a potential health risks to your children.

Hormone residues in beef have been implicated in the early onset of puberty in girls, which could put them at greater risk of developing breast and other forms of cancer, as they grow into adults.

Aside from promoting growth, the routine use of antibiotics is also necessary for preventing disease in animals.

Antibiotics are mixed into the feed of healthy animals in order to prevent disease.

There are now a growing number of shops sprouting throughout the country, selling meat that is free of hormones and antibiotics.

Artificial Coloring
The great bulk of artificial colorings used in food are synthetic dyes. Synthetic food dyes have been implicated to be carcinogenic and many have been banned. Whenever possible, choose foods without dyes.

Preservatives
Nitrite is used as a preservative to preserve meat and helps to prevent the development of off-flavors in cured meat during storage. Nitrite is used in cured meat to inhibit spoilage by microorganisms.

Nitrite has long been suspected as being a cause of stomach cancer. It becomes harmful when food containing nitrites are fried at high temperature. Look for nitrite-free processed meats, better frozen as refrigeration reduces the need for nitrites.

Sulfites
Sulfites are a class of chemicals that can keep cut fruits and vegetables looking fresh. They also prevent discoloration in apricots, raisins, and other dried fruits; control "black spot" in freshly caught shrimp; and prevent discoloration, bacterial growth, and fermentation in wine. It is dangerous to asthmatics.

Artificial Flavoring
Early in this century, a Japanese chemist identified MSG as the substance in certain seasonings that added to the flavor of protein-containing foods. Unfortunately, too much MSG can lead to headaches, tightness in the chest, and a burning sensation in the forearms and the back of the neck. If you think your children are sensitive to MSG, learn to read food labels.

Chemicals in fish

The cleanest fish are the smaller ones, such as anchovies, sardines and mackerel. The larger fish have lived longer and have had more time and space to accumulate pesticide and heavy metal residues including mercury, PCBs and dioxins. Always buy wild fish over farmed fish to avoid antibiotic overloads.

Chemicals in water

Use purified or filtered drinking water. Most unpurified water contains a variety of chemicals that may have a negative impact on the health of your child. Purchase a quality water purifier to overcome this problem.

HOUSEHOLD CHEMICALS

Here is short list some of the most hazardous cleaning products found around the house:

Air Fresheners: Known toxic chemicals found in an air freshener are formaldehyde, a highly toxic, known carcinogen, and phenol.

Carpet and Upholstery Shampoo: Most formulas use highly toxic substances. Some of the chemical contents are cancer causing and can irritate eyes, skin and the respiratory passages.

Dishwasher Detergents: Most products contain chlorine. Each time you wash your dishes, some residue is left on them, which accumulates with each washing. Your food picks up part of the residue especially if your meal is hot.

Furniture Polish: Contain petroleum distillates, which are highly flammable and can cause skin and lung cancer. They contain nitrobenzene, which is easily absorbed through the skin and extremely toxic.

Laundry Products: Laundry detergents contain chemicals such as phosphorus, enzymes, ammonia, naphthalene, phenol, and many others. These substances can cause rashes, itches, allergies, sinus problems and more.

Oven Cleaner: One of the most toxic products people use. They contain lye and ammonia, which harm the skin, and the fumes can affect the respiratory system. Use sea salt and baking soda instead.

Toilet Bowl Cleaners: Usually contain hydrochloric acid, a highly corrosive irritant to both skin and eyes. They also contain hypochlorite bleach, a corrosive irritant that can burn eyes, skin and respiratory tract. Toilet bowl cleaners also may cause pulmonary edema, vomiting or coma if ingested.

Shampoo: When you wash their hair, body and hands, you do so with the intent of killing germs, removing dirt, feeling clean, refreshed and, of course, hygienic. Ironically, some of the very soaps and shampoos such as baby bath, baby lotion, and baby powder that we use to keep the body free of bacteria, dirt and other undesirables; can be extremely toxic to the health of your children.

CHEMICAL IN TOYS

Phthalates are a family of chemicals that are put into plastic baby products such as toys, teething rings and rattles to make them soft and pliable. Phthalates can cause health issues particularly to infants and young children.

Prolonged exposure to toys containing chemicals can greatly affect your children's health and growth. "We've learned the hard way that even small amounts of chemicals can have a negative impact on a child's ability to reach his or her full potential. The well-being of your children is simply too important to ignore," said State Representative Dian Slavens

(D-Canton).

REDUCE EXPOSURE

If you value the health of your children you need to look for ways to reduce or eliminate the use of toxic chemicals in your home and food. Here are some suggestions you can put into practice:

Chemicals At Home

- Buy eco-friendly products such as oils made from citrus, seed, vegetable or pine. By doing so, you are selecting products that are biodegradable and generally less toxic.

- Reduce or eliminate the use of plastics in your home. Plastic wraps, plastic food containers and drink containers contain Bisphenol A (BPA) and other chemicals that are cancer causing. Instead choose glass for storage of food and for reheating and cooking of food.

- Choose pump spray containers instead of aerosols. Pressurized aerosol products often produce a finer mist that is more easily inhaled. Aerosols also put unnecessary volatile organic chemicals into your indoor air when you use them.

- Purchase mercury-free fever thermometer. Use eye drops, contact lens solutions, and nasal sprays and drops that are free of mercury containing preservatives. Exposure to mercury can damage the nervous system, causing problems with thinking, impaired memory, mood, motor skills and problems processing information.

- Vacuum your carpets and floors regularly. Use baking soda, vinegar, or plant-based soaps and detergents to clean your carpet or other surfaces.

- Clean sinks clean sinks, tubs and toilets with baking soda.

- Use vegetable oil with lemon juice to upkeep your wood furniture. Use vinegar and water in a pump spray bottle for cleaning mirrors and shining chrome.

- Use reusable unbleached cotton towels, rags, and non-scratch scrubbing sponges for all-purpose cleaning instead of bleached disposable paper products.

- Use dishwasher detergents that are free of chlorine bleach and lowest in phosphates.

- Use bathroom cleaners that are free of aerosol propellants and antibacterial agents.

Chemicals in Food

- Choose organic fruits and vegetables for your family whenever possible. They have been shown to have less pesticide residue.

- Rinse all fruits and vegetables thoroughly to remove fertilizer residues.

- Don't microwave foods in plastic containers. Chemicals from the plastic container can become absorbed by food during micro-waving.

CLOSING

We live in a world of chemicals. It is almost impossible today to avoid chemicals in your daily life. Your food chain, cooking utensils, drinking containers such as plastic bottles, your household and cleaning products, all contain chemicals that are unhealthy to health.

Make an effort to use eco-friendly alternatives products whenever possible. Toys from wood, cloth, natural fibers and paper are better choices for children than plastic toys. Go organic, especially your vegetables and reduce your children's intake of processed foods which contain preservatives, coloring and flavoring.

Chapter 14

Keep Away From Alcohol, Smoking and Doing Drugs

From time to time, find opportunities to talk to your children about the evils of smoking, drinking or doing drugs. This is important, as they grow older, peer pressure and their increasing need for independence may make them want to defy you.

Most young children are often willing to talk openly to their parents about these controversial subjects; as they are already exposed to these issues daily through the various mass media.

Acknowledge that drugs, alcohol and tobacco are for real and that many people become addicted to them. Patiently explain to them about the long-and short-term effects and its consequences, and the harm it can bring to their growing bodies. Poorly informed children are at greater risk of engaging in and experimenting with alcohol, smoking and drugs.

Don't be judgmental when responding to difficult questions from your child. Keep calm during the discussion and use simple language that your child can understand. Do encourage them to talk about their feelings and their concerns. Make your child feel accepted and respected as an individual by showing them your concern about their health.

Avoid using disciplinary methods such as excessive preaching and threats. Teach your child that freedom only comes with responsibility. This move will increase the chances that your child will try to be open with you.

Set a good example for your children to follow. Don't drink or smoke and do drugs in front of them or have cigarettes, alcohol beverages or drugs lying around the house. Walk the talk. As your child grows into a teenager, he will have the discipline not to fall into the trap of cigarette, alcohol and drug abuse.

As your child grows into a teenager, he or she should have been exposed to your positive attitudes and beliefs about alcohol, smoking and doing drugs. So you can use this time to reinforce what you've already taught your child earlier.

Chapter 15

In a Nutshell

P arents: The health of your children is in your hands. Do not abdicate this responsibility to someone else. It is in the interest of parents to guide their children on how to lead a healthy lifestyle during their *formative years*, as most of the lifestyle diseases such as obesity, diabetes, high blood pressure cancer, heart attacks and strokes have their roots in childhood.

The diets and lifestyle compared to our ancestors have changed drastically. As parents, you need to adjust to these changes if we want to bring up healthy active disease free kids. What are some of the unhealthy changes?

Your diets have gone from fresh food to over-processed, grease-soaked, and laden with chemical, salt and sugar.

Your children's unhealthy eating habits and lifestyle are profoundly influenced from young by advertisements they see on television, the internet, news media, billboard, flyers and magazines. Their lives are surrounded by fast-food outlets, vending machines for fizzy drinks and junky snacks and highly processed foods. Today many children lead sedentary lives. According to US Surgeon General David Satcher in 2001, "This is probably the most sedentary generation of people in the history of the world."

They prefer to spend their free time watching TV,

surfing the net, chatting on their digital hand phones or sending SMS to their friends, playing interactive computer games or listening to music on their ipod.

Many schools around the country are placing priority on academic performance over physical activities. This deprives many children of their most reliable source of exercise.

Today our children are exposed to chronic stress at a young tender age. Pressure of school work, sitting for exams, relocating, abuse parents and peers, starting school or childcare are some examples of stressors. It is important to teach them the ill effects of stress and how to handle them as young as possible as research shows that your child's personality is formed within the first five years.

Many hazardous chemicals are found in our homes and they are toxic to the health of our children. These toxic chemical are harmful to children because of their immature immune system.

Many chemicals exist in our foods such as additives, preservatives, coloring, antibiotics and hormones in animal products of which the long term effect on your children's health is unknown.

Chemicals are also present in our household and cleaning products such as laundry products, oven and toilet bowl cleaners, shampoo. Even their toys, drinking containers such as plastic bottles are not spared. The long-term effects of these chemicals on your children's health is not well researched.

What You Can Do As Parents?

As parents, you need to face the unhealthy challenges that confront the health of your children. To bring up healthy active kids you need to:

• Foster healthy eating habits from young

• Get them to exercise

• Teach them to manage stress

- Teach them that drinking alcohol, smoking and doing drugs are unhealthy practices

- Get your children to go for a routine medical check, five yearly, until they are 20

- Reduce their exposure to household and environmental toxins

- Educate them on lifestyle diseases

- Make sure they drink enough water daily and pay more attention to their sugar, salt and fat intake

- Supplement their diets. Food supplements are not a substitute or excuse for poor dietary choices. For many children, food supplements are no longer an option but a necessity in our toxic environment.

The health of your children is your responsibility. What you do for them today will determine the status of their health as they grow to adulthood.

OVERALL GOLD NUGGETS

"Most progressive doctors are paying close attention to the nutritional and lifestyle habits of their patients and are making sincere recommendations for their patients to stop indulging in tobacco, coffee, and alcohol; to lose excess weight; to exercise moderately; and to follow a low fat, no cholesterol diet." – John A. McDougall M.D.

"To get rich never risk your health. For it is the truth that health is the wealth of wealth." – Richard Baker.

"Never hurry. Take plenty of exercise. Always be cheerful. Take all the sleep you need. You may expect to be well." – James Freeman Clarke.

"Many people treat their bodies as if they were rented from Hertz – something they are using to get around in but nothing they genuinely care about understanding." – Chungliang Al Huang.

"Not only don't diets work; they're actually designed to fail. It's not you or your lack of will power that's the problem. It's that diets by their very nature simply don't work." – Bob Schwartz.

"Your body is a temple, but only if you treat it as one." – Astrid Alauda.

"Water, air, and cleanness are the chief articles in my pharmacy." – Napoleon Bonaparte.

"The desire to take medicine is perhaps the greatest feature which distinguishes man from animals." – Sir William Osler.

"The belly is ungrateful – it always forgets we already gave it something." – Russian Proverb.

"To feel 'fit as a fiddle', you must tone down your middle." – Author unknown.

"No matter who you are, no matter what you do, you absolutely, positively do have the power to change." – Anne Louise Gittleman.

"Genes load the gun, but environment pulls the trigger." – Dr David Herber.

"God heals, and the doctor takes the fee." – Benjamin Franklin.

"Within each of us lies the power of our consent to health and sickness, to riches and poverty, to freedom and to slavery. It is we who control these, and not another." – Richard Bach.

"You can set yourself up to be sick, or you can choose to stay well." – Wayne Dyer.

Bibliography

Book References

Abrahamson, E. and Peget, A. "Body, Mind and Sugar." (New York: Avon, 1977).

Dr. Batmanghelidj. "Your body's many cries for water."

Dufty, William. "Sugar Blues." New York: Warner Books, 1975.

Erasmus U PhD. "Fats that Heal Fats that Kill." Alive Books, 7436 Frazer Park Drive, Burnaby BC, Canada 1996.

Rona, Zoltan P. and Martin, Jeanne Marie. "Return to the Joy of Health, Vancouver." Alive Books, 1995.

Research

Abrahamson, E. and Peget, A. "Body, Mind and Sugar." New York: Avon, 1977.

Albrink, M. and Ullrich I. H. "Interaction of Dietary Sucrose and Fiber on Serum Lipids in Healthy Young Men Fed High Carbohydrate Diets." *American Journal of Clinical Nutrition*, 1986; 43: 419-428. Pamplona, R., et al.

Appelton, Nancy, PhD. "Lick The Sugar Habit." 2nd Edition. Avery, 1988.

Behar, D., et al. "Sugar Challenge Testing with Children Considered Behaviorally Sugar Reactive." *Nutritional Behavior* 1984; 1: 277-288.

Cleave, T. "The Saccharine Disease." *New Canaan*, CT: Keats Publishing, 1974.

Dewailly E, Blanchet C, Lemieux S, et al. "n-3 fatty acids and cardiovascular disease risk factors among the Inuit of Nunavik." *Am J Clin Nutr* 2001; 74(4): 464-473.

Fields, M., et al. "Effect of Copper Deficiency on Metabolism and Mortality in Rats Fed Sucrose or Starch Diets." *Journal of Clinical Nutrition,* 1983; 113: 1335-1345.

Furth, A. and Harding, J. "Why Sugar Is Bad For You." *New Scientist* Sep 23, 1989; 44.

Glinsmann, W., Irausquin, H., and Youngmee, K. "Evaluation of Health Aspects of Sugar Contained in Carbohydrate Sweeteners." *F. D. A. Report of Sugars Task Force* 1986: 39: 00.

Goldman, J., et al. "Behavioral Effects of Sucrose on Preschool Children." *Journal of Abnormal Child Psychology.* 1986; 14(4): 565-577.

Goulart, F. S. "Are You Sugar Smart?" *American Fitness* March - April 1991: 00: 00 34-38. Milwakuee, WI.

Harper CR, Jacobson TA. "The fats of life: the role of omega-3 fatty acids in the prevention of coronary heart disease." *Arch Intern Med* . 2001; 161(18): 2185-2192.

Harris WS. "The omega-6/omega-3 ratio and cardiovascular disease risk: uses and abuses." *Curr Atheroscler Rep.* 2006; 8: 453-459.

Hodges, R., and Rebello, T. "Carbohydrates and Blood Pressure." *Annals of Internal Medicine* 1983: 98: 838-841.

Ludwig, D. S., et al. "High Glycemic Index Foods, Overeating and Obesity." *Pediatrics* March 1999; 103(3): 26-32.

Ludwig D. S., et al. "Relationship between sugar-sweetened drinks and childhood obesity: A prospective, observational analysis." *The Lancet* February 17, 2001, 357 (925): 505-508.

Newton, Ian S. "Long-chain fatty acids in health and nutrition." Business Development, Human Nutrition Department, Roche Vitamins Inc., Parsippany, NJ, USA. ACS Symposium Series (2001), 788 (Omega-3 Fatty Acids), 14-27.

Pennington, Neil L. and Charles Baker, eds. "Sugar: A Users' Guide to Sucrose." Van Nostrand Reinhold, 1991.

Position of the American Dietetic Association: "Nutritive and non-nutritive sweeteners." *Journal of the American Dietetic Association* 2004; 104: 256.

Reiser, S. "Effects of Dietary Sugars on Metabolic Risk Factors Associated with Heart Disease." *Nutritional Health* 1985; 203-216.

Sugano, Michihiro. "Balanced intake of polyunsaturated fatty acids for health benefits." Faculty of Environmental and

Symbiotic Sciences, Prefectural University of Kumamoto, Kumamoto, Japan. *Journal of Oleo Science* (2001), 50(5), 305-311.

Wolever, T.M.S., et. al. "Sugar Alcohols and Diabetes: A Review." *Canadian Journal of Diabetes* 2002; 26: 356.

Yudkin, J., Kang, S. and Bruckdorfer, K. "Effects of High Dietary Sugar." *British Journal of Medicine* Nov 22, 1980; 1396.

Yudkin, J. "Metabolic Changes Induced by Sugar in Relation to Coronary Heart Disease and Diabetes." *Nutrition and Health* 1987; 5(1-2): 5-8.

Glossary

Aerobic Exercise: It is anything that makes you breathe a bit more heavily and increase the pulse rate.

Anaerobic Exercise: Anaerobic exercise help build muscle mass. Strength training is one of the best ways to replace the lean muscle mass that you've lost. Examples of anaerobic exercise include lifting light weights, running short sprints, resistance or interval training.

Aneurysm: A localized "ballooning-out" of the wall of a blood vessel. The increased pressure in the blood vessel coupled with a weakened wall results in aneurysm. An aneurysm may rupture and cause fatal hemorrhages.

Antioxidant: It is a group of compounds found in our body and food that protect the healthy cells and tissues of the body from damage caused by free radicals.

Apple-shaped: People who store excessive body fat around their waists or abdomen are considered to be apple-shaped because, like the fruit, they're largest around the middle.

Artery: A large blood vessel that carries blood from the heart to other parts of the body. Arteries are thicker and have walls that are stronger and more elastic than the walls of veins.

Artificial Sweeteners: The alternative to using a natural or refined sugar; often referred to as non-nutritive sweeteners or sugar substitutes. These sweeteners allow people with weight issues to enjoy a wider variety of foods, in larger servings.

Beta Cells: A type of cell in the pancreas that makes and releases insulin to control the level of glucose (sugar) in the blood. Within the pancreas, the beta cells are located in areas called the Isles of Langerhans.

Blood Clot: Blood that has been converted from a liquid to a solid state.

Blood Glucose: This is main sugar that the body makes from your food intake. Glucose is the major source of energy for living cells and is carried to each cell through the bloodstream. Cells cannot use glucose for energy without the help of insulin.

Blood Vessels: Tubes that carry blood to and from all parts of the body. The three main types of blood vessels are arteries, veins, and capillaries.

Body Mass Index: It is a simple weight-to-height ratio. BMI is a reliable indicator of your total body fat. To calculate your BMI divide your weight by your height squared.

Calorie: The unit of heat energy required to raise 1 kilogram of water one degree Celsius.

Carbohydrates: Carbohydrates are a storage form of sugar.

Cardiovascular Disease: Disease of the heart and blood vessels (arteries, veins, and capillaries).

Cholesterol: An odorless, white, powdery fatty substance similar to fat produced by the liver and found in the blood. It is also found in some foods. Cholesterol is used by the body to make hormones and build cell walls. An elevated level of blood cholesterol is a major cause of coronary heart disease.

Clinical Trials: Trials to evaluate the effectiveness and safety of medications or medical devices by monitoring their effects on large groups of people.

Congestive Heart Failure: Loss of the heart's pumping power, which causes fluids to collect in the body resulting in shortness of breath and chronic coughing.

Conjugated Linoleic Acid (CLA): It is an essential omega-6 fatty acid that the body needs for health but cannot produce on its own. CLA is widely sold commercially as a dietary supplement to aid weight loss by helping to reduce body fat and increase muscle tissue.

Coronary Heart Disease: This disease is caused by narrowing of the arteries that supply blood to the heart mainly due to cholesterol deposits in the artery walls. If the blood supply is cut off, the result is a heart attack.

Cortisol: Cortisol secreted by the adrenal gland controls our appetite, often making us feel hungry even when we have eaten enough. It also raises blood sugar and insulin levels and results in increased fat deposition mainly in the abdominal or belly region. Over time, constant high levels of cortisol may lead to increasing resistance to insulin.

Diabetes: This condition results when our body cannot use blood glucose as energy because of having too little insulin or the cells being unable to use insulin.

Diastolic Blood Pressure: It is the

pressure when the heart rests.

Fiber: A form of carbohydrate from plants that remains largely undigested. Fibers are either soluble or insoluble in water.

Free Radicals: Are incomplete, unstable molecules which are basic building blocks in nature such as oxygen, fatty acids and amino acids.

Fructo-oligosaccharides (FOS): Fructo-oligosaccharides are non-digestible food components found in garlic, onions, leeks, wheat, bananas, asparagus, and artichokes and many others. They are classified as prebiotics. Prebiotics provide food for friendly bacteria in the gut such as bifido-bacteria and lactobacilli at the expense of the unfriendly bacteria but are indigestible to the human body.

Fructose: A simple sugar found in fruits. Its effect on insulin is lower than that of refined sugar or glucose.

Garcinia Cambogia: Is a small, sweet, tropical fruit, native to South India and Southeast Asia. Garcinia is a citrus fruit like lime or grapefruit. The main component of Garcinia cambogia is HCA (Hydroxy citric acid).

Glucagon: It is a fat releasing hormone. Protein foods stimulate the secretion of glucagon. This hormone is secreted by the alpha cells of the pancreas. When your blood glucose falls too low, the pancreas secretes the hormone glucagon and directs the liver to convert the previously stored fat (glycogen) back into glucose. The result: The storage of glucose stops, fat production stops, and glucose (sugar) is released back into the blood stream.

Glycemic Index: The key to carbohydrate selection is the Glycemic Index. Glycemic Index (GI) is a ranking of how quickly 50 grams of a carbohydrate is converted into glucose and enters the bloodstream and spike insulin levels in the body.

Glycemic Load: The GL takes into account both the rate of release (GI) and the total amount of the carbohydrate in a food or mixed meal. It is thus a measure that incorporates both the quantity and quality of the dietary carbohydrates consumed.

Glycogen: A complex form of glucose that is stored in the liver and muscles to be used to meet energy needs.

Gout: It is a disease that affects

the joints of the big toe, the foot and the thumb. In gout, when a person has too much uric acid, a waste product in the urea, some of it forms uric acid crystals. These crystals can deposit in joints, causing pain.

Heart Attack: A heart attack occurs from the blockage in one of the coronary arteries due to atherosclerosis. The blockage stops the blood supply to the heart muscle. Without the necessary oxygen that comes in the blood, the part affected becomes damaged. Depending upon the severity of the damage, disability or death can result.

Heart Disease: Any disorder that affects the heart.

Heart Failure: Inability of the heart to maintain an adequate output of blood.

High Blood Pressure: Pressure in the arteries is your blood pressure. Blood pressure is read as two numbers: Systolic and diastolic. Systolic pressure is generated when your heart muscle contracts and forcefully sends the blood through the arteries. The diastolic pressure is the remaining pressure in the arteries while the heart is refilling and getting ready to beat again.

Human Growth Hormones: Human Growth Hormone (HGH) is called the master hormone. Growth hormone released during sleep is also important for fat loss.

Hyperlipidemia: An abnormally large amount of lipids (fats) in the circulating blood.

Hypoglycemia: Describes a condition of elevated blood sugar.

Hypothyroidism: This means your thyroid is not making sufficient hormone called thyroxine. The thyroid regulates the body's metabolism to control your weight. If you suffer from hypothyroidism, you need to work harder than those without thyroid disease, to lose weight and to keep their weight under control.

Insulin: The hormone insulin produced by the beta cells of the pancreas shuttle the glucose from the bloodstream into the cells and acts like a key that opens the door to the cell so that it can be converted to energy for the body to use. In addition, insulin also controls the rate at which the liver produces and secretes glucose (broken down from stored glycogen) between meals. As the blood sugar drops, insulin shuts off until it is needed again.

Insulin Resistance: If you have insulin resistance, your body cells no longer respond to insulin's command. This resistance by the cells causes glucose to remain high in the bloodstream. If you have insulin resistance, you will have difficulty losing weight.

L-Carnitine: Is a naturally occurring amino acid but its supply is reduced as we age. L-carnitine is synthesized in the liver and kidneys, from two essential amino acids, lysine and methionine, vitamins B6, C, B3, and the mineral iron.

Leptin: This hormone is mostly secreted by fat cells. It is involved in the regulation of appetite, metabolism and calorie burning. Leptin is the hormone that tells your brain when you're full, when it should start burning up calories and when to create energy for the body to use.

Lipid: A term for fat in the body. Lipids can be broken down by the body and used for energy.

Menopause: The term derives from two Greek words: Mens (monthly) and pause (stop). It accurately means the last menstrual period a woman experiences.

Metabolism: The sum of all the chemical and physiological process by which the body grows and maintains itself and by which it breaks matter down into a new state.

Omega-3 Fatty Acids: Also known as polyunsaturated fatty acids; are essential fatty acids. They are essential to human health but cannot be manufactured by the body and must be obtained from food. Omega-3 fatty acids can be found in fish, such as salmon, tuna, and halibut, other marine life such as algae and nut oils. There are three major types of omega-3 fatty acids that are ingested in foods and used by the body: Alpha-linolenic acid (ALA), eicosapentaenoic acid (EPA), and docosahexaenoic acid (DHA).

Obesity: It is not simply weight gain. It's the accumulation of excess body fat.

Osteoarthritis: It is joint disorder that commonly affects the hands, feet, spine and large weight-bearing joints, such as the hip and knees. Extra weight on our joints can wear away the cartilage of your joints. Cartilage is a protein that serves as a "cushion" between the bones of the joints.

Overweight: A person can be

overweight without being obese but an obese person is always over-weight. Overweight and obesity have only one thing in common: That is excess body weight.

Pancreas: The pancreas is an elongated, tapered gland that is located behind the stomach and secretes digestive enzymes and the hormones insulin and glucagon to regulate the body's main energy source, called glucose (blood sugar), in the bloodstream.

Phytochemicals: Are non-nutritive plant chemicals that have protective or disease preventive properties. Lycopene in tomatoes, isoflavones in soy and flavonoids in fruits are some common examples.

Pre-diabetes: A condition in which blood sugar are higher than normal but not high enough to be classified as diabetes. Other names for diabetes are impaired glucose tolerance and impaired fasting glucose.

Refined Sugars: They are processed sugar from plant sources that have their natural fibers, vitamins, amino acid and minerals stripped off. Not only does it totally lack nutrients, but

refined sugar actually robs your body of vitamins, minerals.

Saturated Fats: They are found in most animal fats. They are usually solid at room temperature and are less susceptible to oxidation. The harder the fat, the more saturated fats it contains. A diet high in saturated fats can increase LDL cholesterol and cause insulin resistance.

Sexual Dysfunction: The consistent inability of men to sustain an erection for sexual intercourse or the inability to achieve ejaculation or both, caused by not enough blood flow to the penis.

Stevia: It is a natural sweetener and is extracted from the leaves of a plant called Stevia Rebaudiana that originated in the rainforests of Paraguay. It is known in South America as the "sweet herb."

Stroke: The death of brain cells due to a lack of oxygen when the blood flow to the brain is impaired by blockage or rupture of an artery to the brain. This may cause loss of ability to speak or to move parts of the body.

Subcutaneous Fat: This is the fat you see around your thighs and hip of overweight people. It is directly beneath the skin and on top of the abdominal muscles and can be easily seen in the form of fat rolls.

Sugar Alcohols: They are a type of carbohydrate. Their structure resembles that of sugar and alcohol. They are not as sweet as sucrose or artificial sweeteners.

Trans Fats: A type of fatty acid produced as a result of hydrogenation which is a chemical process by which hydrogen is used to convert liquid oils into a solid form such as margarine.

Triglyceride: The storage form of fat in the body.

Vein: A blood vessel that carries blood to the heart.

Visceral Fat: Are often found in close contact with subcutaneous fat in the abdominal region. They are unhealthy fats that lie deep in the abdomen beneath your muscle and surround your vital organs such as the heart, liver, kidney, gallbladder and pancreas, putting you at risk of heart disease, insulin resistance and diabetes.

Waist Circumference: It is a measure of abdominal fat and a better indicator of your health status, even when the BMI calculation falls within the range classified as normal.

Waist-to-Hip Ratio: Using a measuring tape to check your hip-to-waist ratio is another way of judging whether your weight is healthy. The waist-to-hip ratio refers to the comparison of weight carried between your waist and hip. Waist-to-hip ratio is a simple measure of where fat is distributed in your body. The waist-to-hip ratio is a measure of abdominal obesity.

Simple books for understanding health

 OAK BETTER HEALTH SERIES

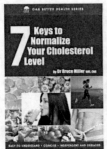

7 Keys to Normalize Your Cholesterol Level
In this book, you will discover seven keys in simple and concise language, you can take to lower your cholesterol to a healthy level.

7 Keys To Bring Your Blood Pressure Under Control
This book gives you seven crucial keys you can take today to lower your blood pressure and keep it under control or prevent it in the first place. Start using these keys today to avoid becoming a candidate for a heart attack or stroke.

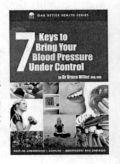

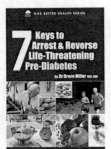

7 Keys to Arrest & Reverse Life-Threatening Pre-Diabetes
This book lays down seven keys to avoid being a victim of full blown diabetes. This will add years to your life and life to your years as pre-diabetes causes heart attack or stroke, two main silent killers of the human race.

7 Keys to Bring Your Diabetes Under Control
Within these easy-to-read pages, you will find seven crucial keys to help you control your sugar level to near normal as possible and improve your cell's sensitivity to insulin to prevent or delay the onset of long-term complications of the disease.

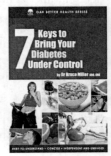